EXERCISES IN DIAGNOSTIC RADIOLOGY

1
THE CHEST

LUCY FRANK SQUIRE, M.D.

Lecturer, Harvard Medical School; Visiting Radiologist,
Massachusetts General Hospital, Boston, Massachusetts

WILLIAM M. COLAIACE, M.D.

Lecturer in Medical Science, Brown University;
Radiologist, Roger Williams General Hospital,
Providence, Rhode Island

NATALIE STRUTYNSKY, M.D.

Assistant Professor, Radiology, New York Medical
College, New York City

W. B. SAUNDERS COMPANY • PHILADELPHIA • LONDON • TORONTO   1970

W. B. Saunders Company: West Washington Square
Philadelphia, Pa. 19105

12 Dyott Street
London, WC1A 1DB

1835 Yonge Street
Toronto 7, Ontario

Exercises in Diagnostic Radiology — Volume I The Chest

Print No.:   9   8   7   6   5   4   3   2   1

PREFACE FOR
STUDENTS AND TEACHERS

We have hesitated to call this a workbook, for the term seems alien to the dignified learning program we would hope to see offered to the graduate students whom we call medical students. We dislike the condescension implied toward the student in much of the programed material we have seen; condescension is no way to make learning palatable. Most medical students are serious young people and do not need to have rote patterns supplied them, but rather learning materials suitable to their stage of information and attractive to them in format. In our opinion they need a larger volume of more straightforward clinical material to study, particularly examples which they are likely to be able to analyze and interpret themselves without much assistance, and mixed in among these a few difficult problems to stimulate reading and stretch the mind.

So here is a little book full of problems, the solving of which should teach radiology while entertaining the reader. This book and those to follow are intended to function late in medical training and during the first year of graduate training as self-testing, self-instructional supplements to *Fundamentals of Roentgenology* (LFS).* The exercises in this first volume on the chest are based on the assumption that *the student will have read the first ten chapters of the textbook.* By expecting the student to have at least that much experience in roentgen diagnosis, we have been able to construct exercises which are neither too simple to be interesting nor uniformly difficult. Alternation of more and less difficult case material allows the student to be stimulated by his mistakes and encouraged by his successes. He will notice this assumption of some experience in radiology has enabled us to put together random case material similar to what one might see on any given night in the Emergency Ward.

The reader would not be entertained by guessing the point of an exercise immediately; that should be evident only as one reviews it after it has been completed and the answers studied. Therefore, students are urged to follow directions closely, and to work through the book from beginning to end. The exercises are progressive and often interlocked. Readers should make a practice of tipping and folding the pages as directed so that PA and lateral films are viewed together as the layout arrangement provides.

---

*Harvard University Press, 1964.

The reader must also be urged to study with a blank tablet at hand on which he writes down his answers before turning to the answer page spread which follows. Long experience with exercises of this sort has shown how much more is learned by such fidelity of purpose.

In addition to the self-testing function of this book, we hope it may serve as an aid to overworked teachers of radiology. Perhaps they will find that the assignment of particular page spreads in class will prepare the way for viewing groups of actual film cases of a similar character.

LUCY FRANK SQUIRE
WILLIAM M. COLAIACE
NATALIE S. STRUTYNSKY

ACKNOWLEDGMENTS

The authors wish to express their gratitude to Drs. Barbara Carter and Jeffery Moore, who have generously supplied us with film case material and financial assistance in the costly preparation of photographic copies of radiographs. Dr. Adele K. Friedman has allowed us to use her collection of material on the acute abdomen, which will appear in the second volume. We are much indebted to Dr. Alice Ettinger, who gave us her valued critical opinion on the manuscript, reflecting her rich experience in teaching undergraduate radiology. For case materials from the Massachusetts General Hospital we thank Dr. Laurence L. Robbins, and for material from St. Luke's Hospital in New York City we thank Dr. Nathaniel Finby. The Harvard Press has kindly allowed us to re-use a few illustrations from the textbook *Fundamentals of Roentgenology*: Figures 3-2 **A** and **B**, 4-15, 8-11, 8-24 **A** and **B**, 8-25 **A** and **B**, 9-5, 9-6, 9-11, **D, E** and **F,** 10-46, 10-49 and 10-50. We also thank Francine Cluxton for hours of coding and filing, and Selma Surman for typing the manuscript. The Eastman Kodak Company, in particular Mr. William Cornwell, gave us invaluable advice before we undertook the project. Finally, we are very much indebted to John Schwartz, presently a fourth year medical student at New York University, who served as a test subject, going through every word of the finished manuscript, writing out his answers to every exercise, and furnishing us with the best imaginable "feedback" on the book from a member of its intended audience. Without his high standards for clarity of purpose in the phrasing of questions and the answers provided we should have been much less willing to release to the publisher this first volume of experimental exercises. We would welcome from readers their ideas, suggestions, criticisms and needs for the future as we prepare the additional volumes.

LUCY FRANK SQUIRE
WILLIAM M. COLAIACE
NATALIE S. STRUTYNSKY

One West Seventy-second Street
New York, New York 10023

Teaching is only guidance toward the excitement of discovery. The problems on the first few page spreads are a review and an amplification of the basic roentgen concepts covered in Chapter 1 of *Fundamentals of Roentgenology* (LFS). Without the logical habits of mind described there you cannot expect to analyze film studies systematically, nor can you anticipate your own capacity for thinking three-dimensionally about roentgen shadows.

Remember three things:

1. Roentgen white-gray-black values are the result of variations in the number of rays which have passed through the object radiographed to blacken the film. They are, therefore, *always* summation shadowgrams of all the masses in the full thickness of the object which has been interposed between beam-source and film.

2. The margin of *any* shadow on the film represents a tangentially seen interface between two masses of different roentgen density (average atomic number determines roentgen density). If one of the two masses changes so that they are alike in density, there will be no differential interface and the shadow margin will disappear.

3. Awareness of the range of atomic numbers (roentgen densities) of objects or tissues plus the information you will deduce about their thickness, shape and form *may* make it possible for you to identify an object by name from its radiograph.

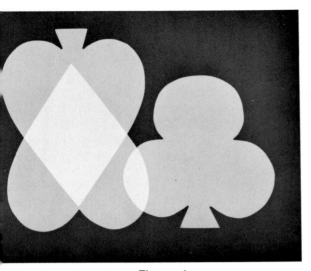

Figure 1

Problem: Is there a diamond in this hand?

Items to decide: Interpret the film as a summation shadowgram. What was the probable composition of the objects interposed between beam source and film? Shape? Thickness? Uniform or varied? Deduce the three-dimensional form and name/identity of the objects radiographed.

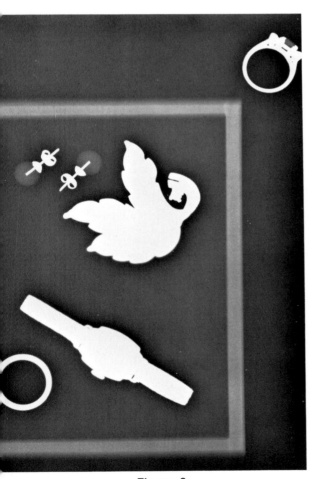

Figure 2

Problem: Account for the shape and form (and if possible identity) of every part of the objects radiographed. Why do the shadows of the objects have margins?

Short cut: Start by allowing intuition to suggest identity and then subject the guess you have made to logical analysis.

ANSWER: There is no diamond present, overlap or "summation" alone accounting for the diamond-shaped, denser area where the pointed ends of the heart and spade have been intentionally superimposed. An ellipse of the same density as the "diamond" is accounted for by overlap of part of the heart and club. From their roentgen shadows you should be able to state with confidence that the three "objects" were thin, metal, of uniform thickness, cut into the shapes of heart, club and spade and radiographed in air. (They were aluminum bridge coasters 3 mm thick.) Summate or overlap them differently and they appear as in Figure 3. Would they disappear if radiographed immersed in a medium composed of minute spherical granules of the same metal in a layer just 3 mm thick? (Answer on opposite page)

A jewel box made of wood with a hinged lid which was closed. Box contained a ring, a brooch, and a pair of (false) pearl earrings for pierced ears. A watch had been laid on top of the box. The ring outside the box had a central

diamond, of good quality, at least according to its owner ... but isn't diamond just compressed carbon? Glass filmed in air should x-ray like this, by the way, but (depending on its mineral content) may have nearly the same density as muscle in which it is embedded after injury. (Felman and Fisher: The radiographic detection of glass in soft tissue. Radiology 92(7): 1529, June, 1969.)

In the space between the images of the watch and the brooch, summate what is actually being radiographed. (Answer on opposite page.)

The margin of any radiographic shadow is produced by a sudden change in the number of rays traversing matter or, in other words, by the existence of a tangentially seen *interface* of some sort between masses of different roentgen density, here metal and air, or wood and air. Think in terms of summation shadows and of interfaces across which x-rays slide tangentially, and you will be able to "account" for any radiographic shadow.

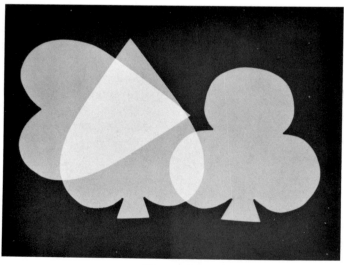

Figure 3

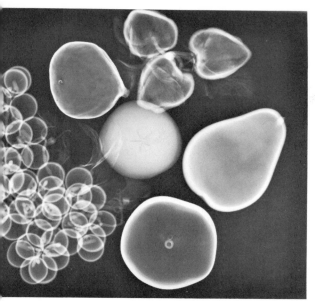

Figure 4

PROBLEMS

Figure 4. Real or artificial fruit? Why? (Analyze each roentgen shadow as composite shadowgram with interfaces.)

Figure 5. Name/identify object radiographed. Justify your conclusion according to the basic principles roentgen shadows obey. By the way, is it "normal" or sick?

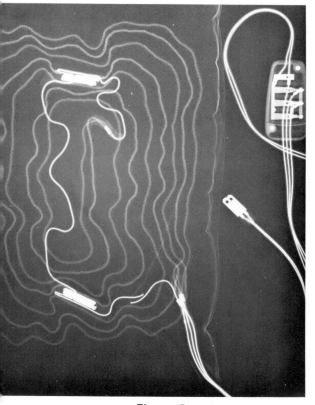

Figure 5

ANSWERS TO QUESTIONS ON PAGE 2
(1) The bridge coasters would be seen faintly.
(2) Top and bottom of box plus air above box and air inside box are being radiographed.

ANSWERS

Figure 4. All fruit was artificial except the central piece, which was an excellent pear. The water-dense meat does not have a different density from the tough skin; the edges are more "radiolucent" because there is less pear there and more rays passed through to blacken the film. The stem is not quite perfectly superimposed on the stellate core and is seen to the left* of it as an extra dense (white) spot because it was *added* to the density of the full thickness of the pear.

The artificial fruit is seen to be hollow, the tangentially filmed shell of each accounting for the ring-like shadow, air within and air without to give you *two* air/plastic interfaces. (What would a real bunch of grapes look like if radiographed?)

Figure 5. A "sick" electric heating pad. It has a fractured wire. There appear to be two sorts of wires because . . . ? (Answer on Page 5.)

---

*The "patient's" left, remember.

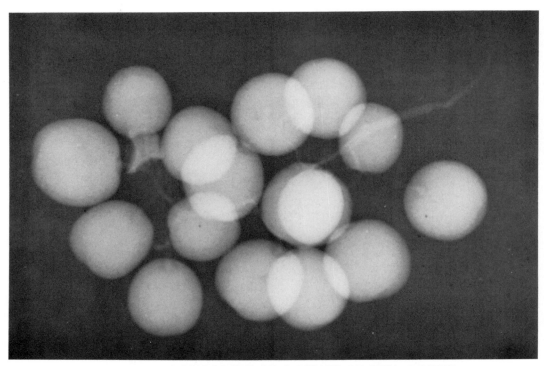

Figure 6   RADIOGRAPH OF A BUNCH OF REAL GRAPES.

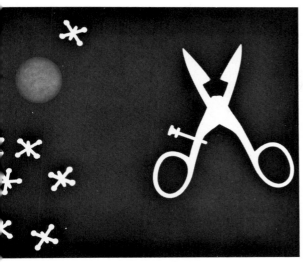

Figure 7

PROBLEM: Can you name/identify the objects which have been radiographed? (Be precise—what *kind* of scissors?)

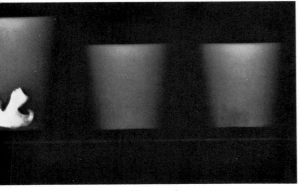

Figure 8

PROBLEM: Paper cups partly filled with water, each containing a block of tissue, were radiographed from the side. What kind of tissue was immersed in water in each cup? Justify all interfaces. (The cups themselves cast no roentgen shadow.)

ADDITIONAL PROBLEMS (NO FIGURES):

Predict precisely (or diagram) the radiograph of a three-inch thick slab of Swiss cheese.

Predict the appearance of a radiograph of a stillborn infant.

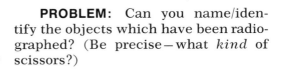

ANSWERS CONTINUED FROM PRECEDING PAGE:
More on heating pad: There are two sorts of electric wires in a heating pad—one a heavy copper wire of large caliber and low resistance and others which are spirals of very fine wire with a high resistance. On the original print the fine spirals could be seen clearly.

ANSWERS

Figure 7. A rubber ball, a set of jacks, and a pair of buttonhole scissors. (The screw in the handle governs the size of the hole cut.) If you failed to identify the scissors, it was probably because you did not know they existed. Neither did I. You cannot expect to identify the radiographic image of an object you have no knowledge of, nor can you be expected to figure out the changes in the radiographic appearance of tissues and structures in disease unless you are familiar with the pathology and know how it affects those tissues. (Incidentally, the vital importance of being familiar with objects, form, tissues and pathologic change is well illustrated by the fact that we showed this radiograph to a three-year-old who had watched his mother sewing but had not played with older children. His instant response was, "That is a pair of buttonhole scissors and these are a moon and some stars." All a question of familiarity!)

Figure 8. Chunks of bone, fat, and muscle had been immersed in the water. The bone/water and fat/water interfaces are easy to recognize. The muscle in the center cup is the same density as the water and there is, therefore, no differential interface to outline it. (The fat did not float because it was stuck to the bottom of the cup by the time we got back to the x-ray department.)

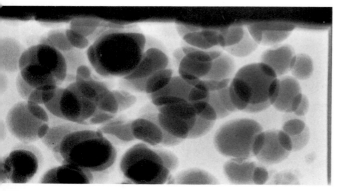

Figure 9

SWISS CHEESE: You probably came close if you decided to think first of the *structure* radiographed — a homogeneous matrix of water-density containing many empty spherical spaces, some of which would overlap others above or below and so produce elliptical areas where more rays would pass through to blacken the film.

Contrast these with the ellipses in Figure 6. (Incidentally, a New York taxi driver, given a little briefing in basic radiology, was able to predict the appearance of this film two hours before it was made.)

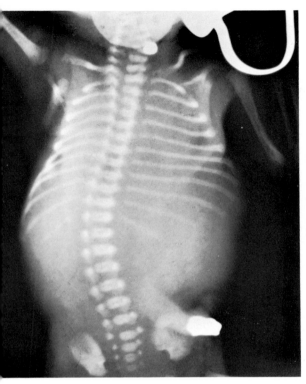

Figure 10

STILLBORN: The stillborn, if he has never expanded his lungs or swallowed air, must be homogeneously water-density from chin to symphysis pubis. Heart, lungs, liver, spleen, and collapsed gut all have the same roentgen density and cast a confluent shadow with no boundary interfaces to outline any of these structures. The slight variations in density over the chest are skin folds.

READ CAREFULLY

From this point on, double page spreads with lettered *problem films,* questions relating to them, and so forth, will alternate with **Answer** page spreads throughout the book. Because I think the student learns more when he has several similar film studies to look at together, each **Problem** page spread will have several films and a number of problems. You should study all the films on the page at once *before* turning to the **Answer** page spread. Employ the corresponding parts and structures of all films on the same page as normals to check what you feel to be abnormal on one film. Be sure that

you have thought through the answer to every question and problem on a **Problem** page spread before turning to the answers, since frequently the problems will be interrelated. One problem may help you with another on the same page. It is, however, anticipated that you will have studied the first ten chapters in *Fundamentals of Roentgenology* before going beyond this point. The self-checking/self-testing procedure for which the workbook is designed will be greatly enhanced and rendered much more interesting to you if you treat each new **Problem** page spread as a group of films on your own patients about which you must reach a decision, unassisted.

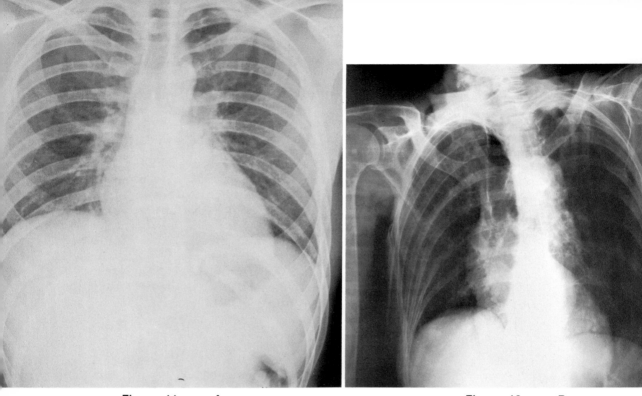

Figure 11   A

Figure 12   B

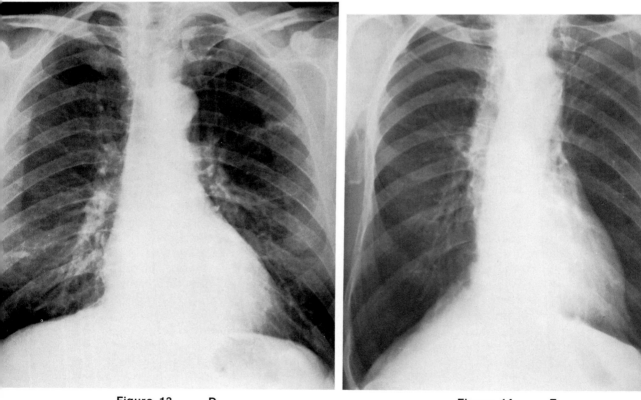

Figure 13   D

Figure 14   E

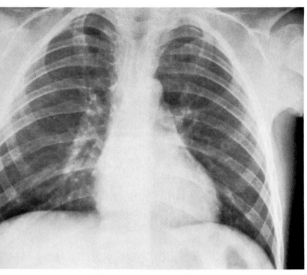

Figure 15   C

Study These Six Chest Films
Systematically

Begin with the six pairs of **Clavicles.**

Are any of these films made with a **Not Perfectly Sagittal Beam?** B

Do any of the **Hearts** appear to be enlarged? F

Make a decision about each of the 12 **Hemidiaphragm Lung Interfaces.**

Identify three undesirable **Technical Imperfections.** How could the technician have avoided them? Were any justifiable, perhaps, in view of the abnormal film findings?

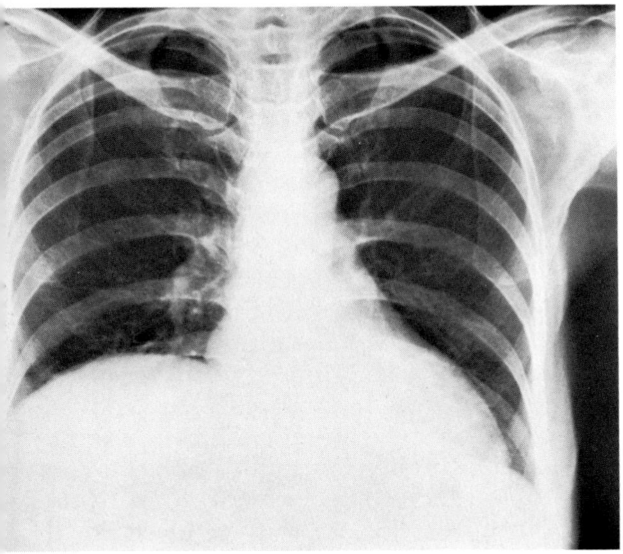

Figure 16   F

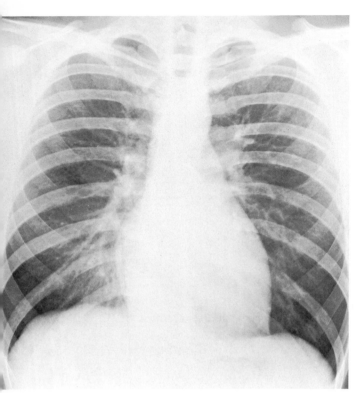

Figure 17   **GOES WITH A**

ANSWERS

Clavicles are normal in **A, E,** and **F** but asymmetrical in **B,** which indicates that the patient was rotated off the sagittal plane. **D** shows a fresh fracture of the left clavicle with overriding. **C** has no clavicles, or at least only fragmentary ribbons of bone where they should be, a congenital defect.

All except **B** are made with a perfectly **Sagittal Beam.** Note how precisely the medial ends of the clavicles center on the white teardrop representing the spinous process of T3 in **F.** The patient in **B** was an elderly woman unable to stand and radiographed with great difficulty in her bed. Because of rotation and projection, her heart appears enlarged and her mediastinum widened.

Diaphragmatic Interfaces are seen at expiration in **A;** are normal in **B, C,** and **D;** are low, flat and fixed at fluoroscopy in **E,** an old gentleman who had emphysema clinically. The high right diaphragm in **F** was due to a very large liver full of metastases from a carcinoma of the colon. (Note Figure 19, the related lateral.)

Hearts: A's heart might appear to be borderline enlarged, but the diaphragms are high (rib 9) and this is therefore a poor inspiration film. Figure 17 is a film made on the same patient with a good inspiration.

Technical Imperfections: A, made at expiration, was repeated at inspiration. **B** is overexposed and was not made with a sagittal beam, but the lung fields appeared clear of important pneumonic change when the film was bright-lighted, and since the patient was in great pain from a ureteral calculus, repetition of the film was felt to be unnecessary by both internist and radiologist. **A,B,D,E,** and **F** all show scapulae overlying the upper lung field, which may usually be avoided by rotating the shoulders forward. In none of these patients was it thought to be important enough to warrant repeating the film. In Patient **D,** it could not have been done anyway because of pain in the fractured clavicle.

THE LATERAL CHEST FILM

Most people find the lateral chest film a difficult muddle. There is no need to if you approach it systematically. Start with the **Two Diaphragmatic Outlines.** The right usually appears as a clean sharp interface (lung/liver) extending from the low, pointed posterior sulcus straight forward to the anterior chest wall. The left extends forward only to the back of the cardiac shadow where the heart sits on the anterior part of the left diaphragm. The interface disappears from this point forward because the roentgen density of the left lobe of the liver and of the heart is the same.

Make a systematic visual inspection of the **Two Posterior Sulci,** almost but not exactly superimposed in Figure 18. In Figure 19 the right is much higher than the left because of the large liver beneath the diaphragm.

Now look at the thoracic vertebrae from top to bottom. Check the density of the vertebrae on every lateral chest film since ill-defined densities in the posterior part of either lung will increase the whiteness of the vertebrae, a simple summation like that of the big liver in Figure 19.

The shadow of the **Heart** is well anterior in the chest. In front of the heart and behind the heart are the **Anterior and Posterior Clear Spaces,** radiolucent areas where the two lungs often touch, which should be checked because either may contain masses and so become dense.

Check the **Air Shadow of the Trachea.** The superimposed branching **Hilar Vessels** lie below it.

Now that you have studied the lateral chest systematically, you should be able to "account for" that large, dense, white wedge overlying the lower part of the heart in Figure 19. It can be "summated" as "carcinoma-filled liver plus heart plus breast." Did you note that the patient in Figure 18 is a male and the one in Figure 19 a female?

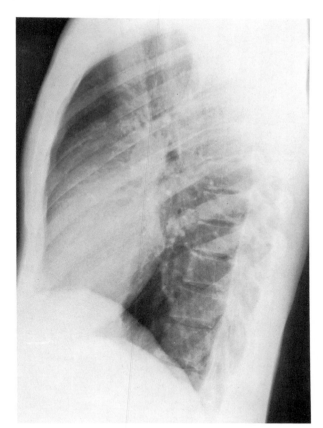

Figure 18   GOES WITH A

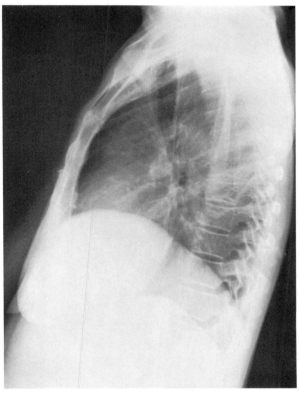

Figure 19   GOES WITH F

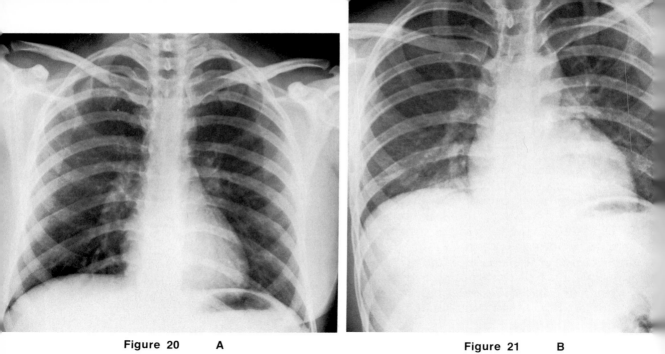

Figure 20   A

Figure 21   B

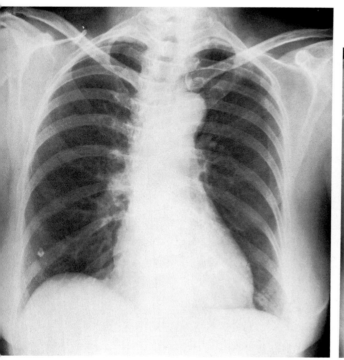

Figure 22   D

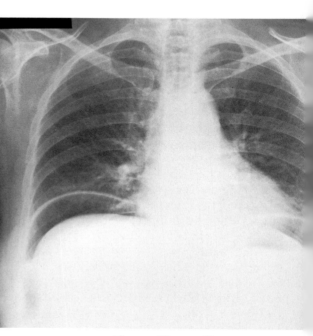

Figure 23   E

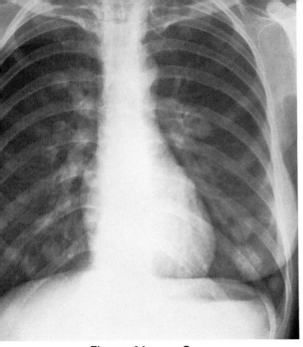

Figure 24   C

Study and Analyze Systematically These Six Patients

Which films can you be absolutely certain were taken standing?

Do you think any of these people have cardiac enlargement?

Would you have any films repeated?

How many women are there among the six?

One patient fell off a horse last week — which one?

One of these patients had major surgery a year ago and one will have surgery this afternoon — which?

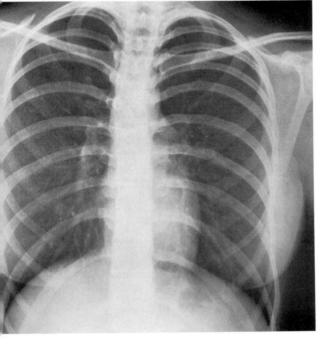

Figure 25   F

ANSWERS

Patients **A,B,C,** and **E** are **Standing** because there are fluid levels where the ray slides tangentially across an interface between air and gastric contents. In addition, the patient in **E** has fluid/air interfaces at both sides of the upper abdomen which are too close to the lateral abdominal wall to be intraluminal. These tell you that the patient has free air and fluid in the peritoneal space. She was a middle-aged woman sitting quietly in clinic, having had an appointment for ten days to "see about" her recurrent ulcer symptoms. Note the interface which represents the outside of the gastric fundus outlined by free air under the left diaphragm. Figure 30 is her lateral film.

B and **E** are poor inspiration films. **Repeat** film **B** (see Figure 26). There is no time and no need to repeat **E.**

All were **Women** except **B,** a young man whose gastric fluid level on this occasion was a CO_2/Pepsi-Cola interface. The breasts in **E** were heavy and pendulous and hard to see on either the **PA** or the lateral view.

Unanswerable question: The woman you see in **D** actually did **Fall off a Horse** last week, but she had nothing to show for it but bruises. Her chest film did show a small calcification in the lower right lung field, but it proved to be in the breast rather than in the lung (see lateral Figure 27) and had nothing to do with the trauma. Patient **A** has an old well-healed fracture of her left clavicle.

SURGERY: The patient in **C** had a radical mastectomy a year ago and now has multiple round pulmonary metastases. Contrast the high arched soft tissue of skin fold on the right, where breast and pectoral muscles have been removed, with the gentle curve on the left, where the axillary fold joins the remaining breast. The patient in **E** had emergency surgery as soon as it could be arranged that afternoon, the

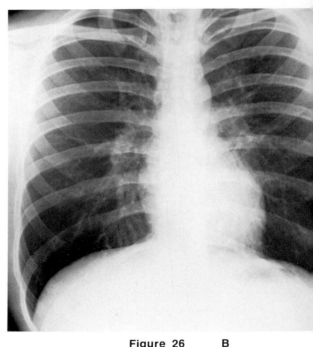

Figure 26   B

perforated ulcer was repaired, and she made a good recovery.

F is a normal chest film and Figure 28 is that patient's lateral.

NOTE: The occasional interpolation of **Normal Films** throughout the workbook is intended to enhance your enjoyment of the exercises, and, after all, more nearly corresponds to the assortment of film problems common to your professional workday. The automatic bias with which we all approach the usual CPC exercise decreases its meaningfulness as an inducement to think sensibly.

Use page 15 as a review exercise in analyzing the lateral chest film. (But beware the garden path!)

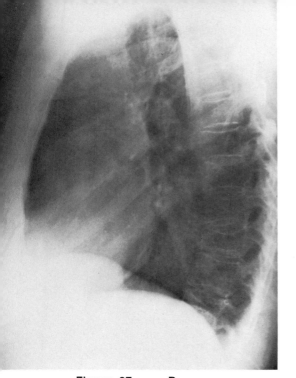

Figure 27   D

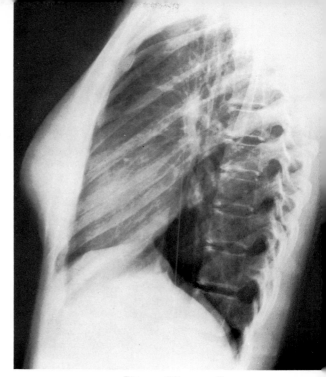

Figure 28   F

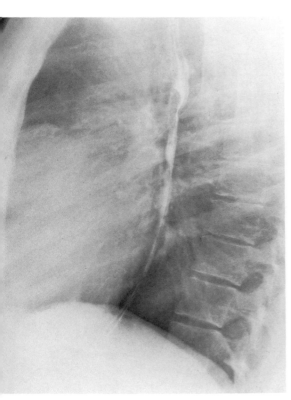

Figure 29   ?

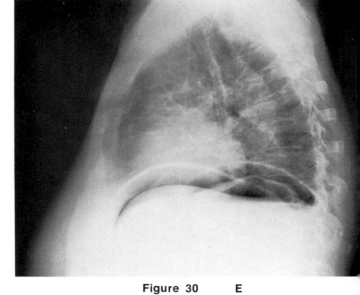

Figure 30   E

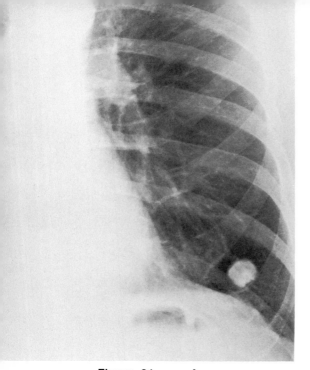

Figure 31　　A

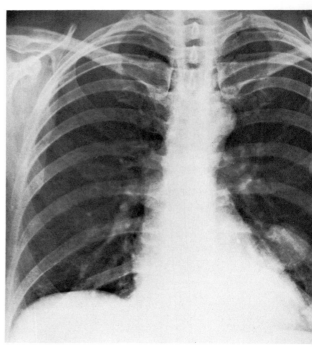

Figure 32　　B

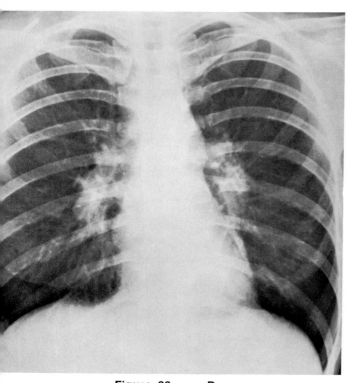

Figure 33　　D

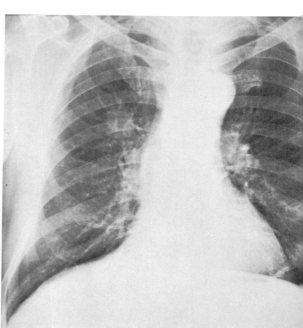

Figure 34　　E

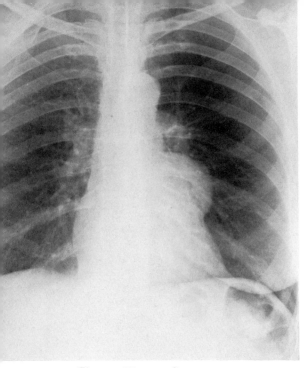

Figure 35   **C**

These six patients were entirely asymptomatic. Examine their chest films as you would if they had come to you for an annual check-up. All were within a year or so of age 40 except **E**, who was 57.

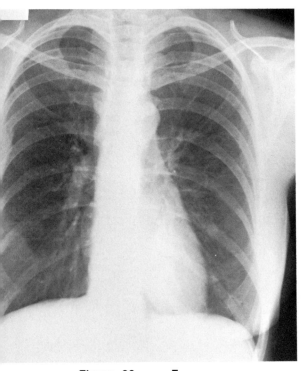

Figure 36   **F**

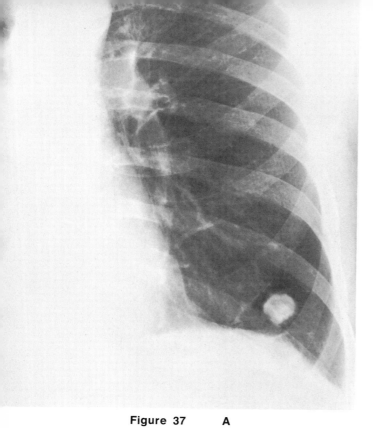

Figure 37   **A**

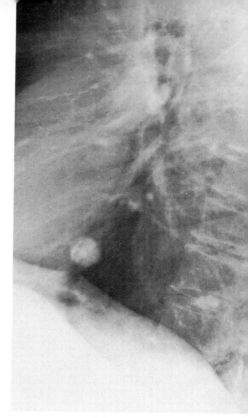

Figure 38   **A**

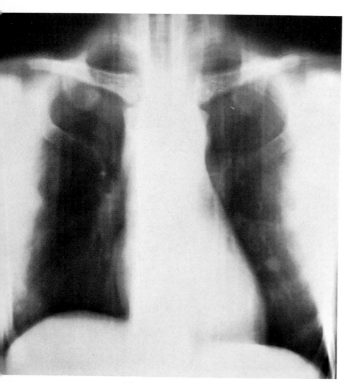

Figure 39   **F**

ANSWERS

Patient A has a solitary spheroid mass in the left lower lung field. It is so dense that one must conclude that it has calcium throughout. The mere presence of calcium, although more likely to indicate an inflammatory lesion, does not exclude the possibility of a neoplasm which has engulfed an earlier granuloma. However, the calcium in this lesion is so diffusely distributed that malignancy is practically ruled out. Figure 37 shows the same lesion a year later, unchanged, and Figure 38 is the patient's lateral film. A less strikingly calcified solitary mass would probably be resected in most clinics today in a shorter period than a year.

NOTE: None of the usually quoted roentgen criteria for deciding the character of a solitary lesion can be absolutely depended upon. Neither minor calcification, nor secondary satellites, nor slow growth rate *proves* benignity; neither umbilication nor ray formation *proves* malignancy.

Patient B was found at surgery to have an adenocarcinoma, not visible at bronchoscopy and located far posteriorly against the chest wall.

Patient C has a bulge too abrupt in its takeoff from the cardiac shadow to be probably vascular in character. It is true that angiocardiography would establish for you whether this is a non-vascular mass, but you have already seen this patient's lateral film (Figure 29; look again). This is a mass in the anterior mediastinum which you may have noted for the reason that the lower part of the anterior clear space contained something with a sharp upper interface border. The patient had subclinical symptoms of myasthenia gravis (occasional double vision when fatigued). A thymoma was removed surgically.

Patient D has bilateral hilar nodes and paratracheal nodal masses which widen the mediastinal shadow. This was a pre-employment chest film and the patient proved to have sarcoidosis on biopsy of a peripheral node. Note the radiolucent space between heart and nodes often seen in sarcoidosis since the nodes are actually intrapulmonary and peribronchial rather than strictly hilar.

This is not true of **Patient E.** He does have hilar nodes, though they are much less striking. He also has a very low-density, solitary nodule overlying the right seventh rib near the spine which proved at autopsy a few days later to be a primary bronchogenic carcinoma. The patient died from hemorrhage into unsuspected cerebral metastases. Note the irregular calcification in the first rib cartilages, which is normal and quite common.

No, **Patient F** does not have a normal chest film. There is a denser spot where the posterior ninth rib on the left crosses the anterior part of the fourth. This spot is suspiciously more dense than any other rib crossing. Figure 39 on this page spread is a laminagram confirming the presence of the small 1-cm. carcinoma, which was resected at surgery. Perhaps the other patients in this group with solitary lesions raised your index of suspicion, but will you spot the next very small carcinoma in a salvageable, asymptomatic patient?

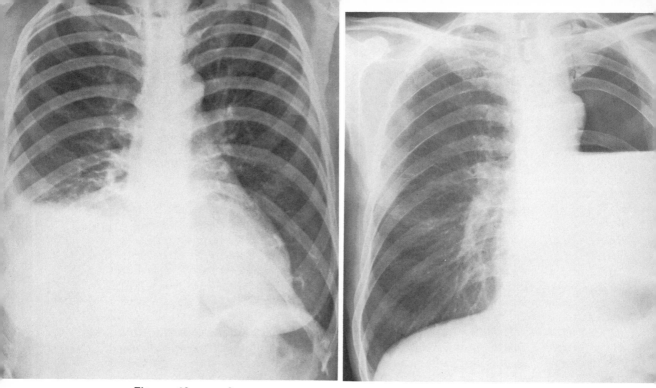

Figure 40   A

Figure 41   B

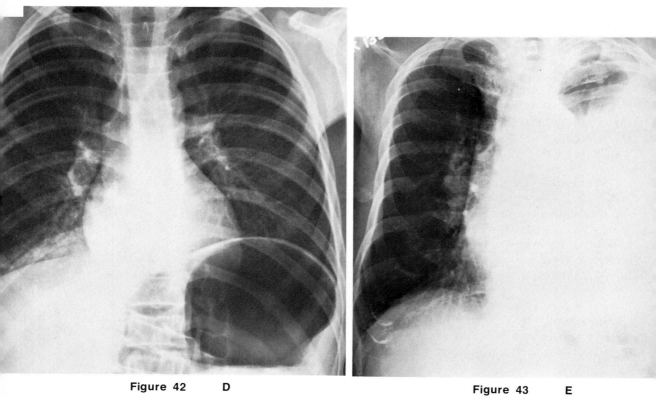

Figure 42   D

Figure 43   E

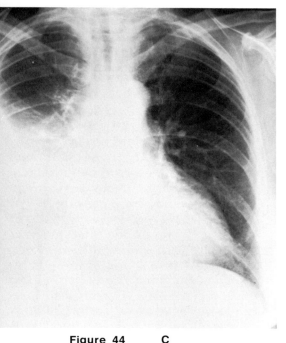

Figure 44   **C**

PROBLEMS

Check these six films for rotation and for degree of inspiration. All six patients had **Dyspnea** and **Chest Pain**. **A** and **D** had fever. Anticipate the roentgen shadows on the lateral chest films in **A,B,C,** and **D.**

Is there a valid **Mediastinal Shift** in any of these films?

How many have **Pleural Effusion**?

Has any of these patients roentgen evidence of **Previous Surgery,** recent or remote?

On which would you want supplementary film studies? Anticipate the appearance of the ones you request.

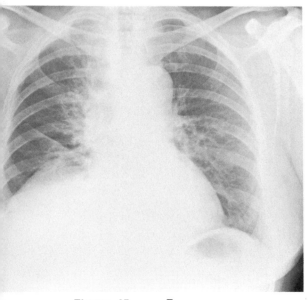

Figure 45   **F**

WHEN STUDYING ANSWERS PLACE EDGE OF PAGE 22 IN CENTER OF PAGE 20 IN ORDER TO VIEW PA FILM AND RELATED LATERAL ON THE SAME PATIENT TOGETHER. THIS ARRANGEMENT FOR VIEWING IS SET UP THROUGHOUT THE BOOK.

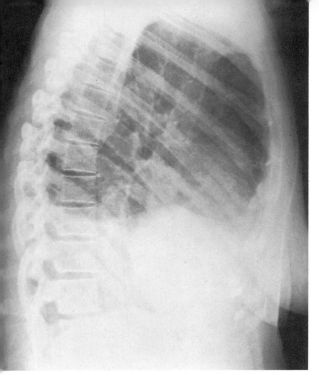

Figure 46   A

ANSWERS

All the films are made with a sagittal beam; none is rotated.

All six films were made at **Deep Inspiration for That Patient.** There is, therefore, no point in repeating any of these films. Note that in **A,** although the right diaphragmatic leaf is at the tenth rib, the left leaf has been pulled down almost to the twelfth. In each patient one of the two diaphragms is obscured or high but you can estimate inspiratory effort from the other.

One would request lateral films on **A,D,** and **F,** hoping for more information about the posterior sulci and lower lung fields. In **B,C,** and **E** there is not much to be gained from a lateral film since the pleural effusion is so large that it will obscure other film findings. Figure 50 is the related lateral to **B.** The patient had had a left pneumonectomy a few days before and has the expected hydropneumothorax.

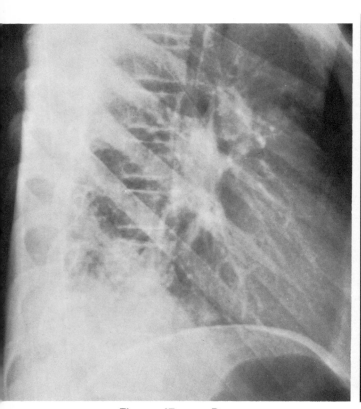

Figure 47   D

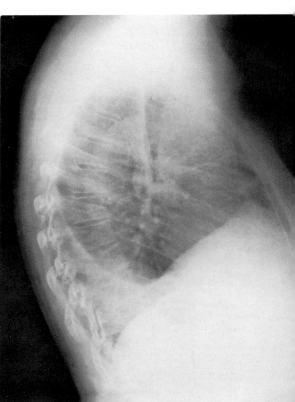

Figure 48   F

In **A** *some* fluid in the right sinus together with a high "diaphragm" suggests infrapulmonary fluid. Figure 46 shows fluid in one posterior sulcus. In the **Lateral Decubitus Film** (Fig. 49) the fluid has been dumped out and lies against the lateral chest wall.

NOTE: The normal lower right lung may now be seen. The white triangle over the heart is a summation of heart plus breast.

Patient **D** had a right **Lower Lobe Pneumonia,** seen near the heart and just above the diaphragm. In the lateral film (Fig. 47) only one diaphragm is visible, the left, outlined from both sides by air. The right diaphragmatic interface has disappeared posteriorly because of the confluence of pneumonic lung and liver shadow.

With regard to **Mediastinal Shift,** remember that the normal location for the trachea is in the midline down to the clavicles and then displaced slightly to the right by the arch of the aorta. In **B** it is shifted slightly *toward* the side of the effusion; a whole lung is missing and the volume of the hydropneumothorax may not exactly equal the volume of the right lung. The normal course postpneumonectomy is for the mediastinum to shift gradually farther and farther to the side of the missing lung as air and fluid are resorbed until the pleural space is obliterated and the heart lies against the chest wall. The appearance of the chest film will then almost exactly resemble that for total collapse of one lung.

The lower trachea and right heart shadow in patient **E** *are* shifted to the right by this very large effusion. In **C, E,** and **F** the effusion was due to malignant seeding of the pleura. (What! You hadn't noticed the missing right breast in **F**?) Much of the fluid in **F** is infrapulmonary and some is probably loculated in the fissures by new growth.

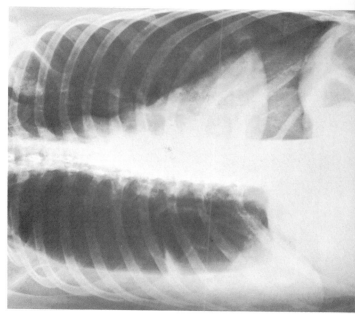

Figure 49   **A**

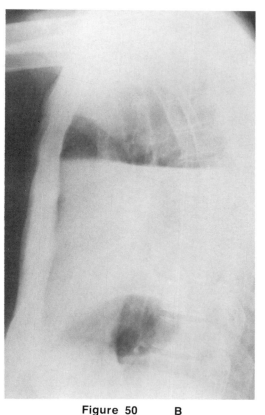

Figure 50   **B**

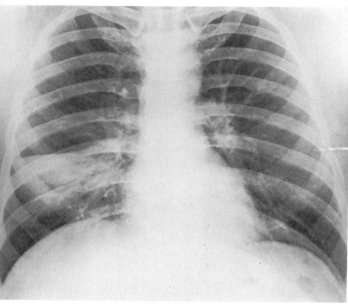

Figure 51   **BILL DEAN**

PROBLEMS

It is your evening on duty in the emergency division. You see these four patients within two hours.

Bill Dean and Ann Pulsifer, both under 25, complain of **Chest Pain, Fever, and Cough** for about 48 hours. Both were well a week ago. You do careful physical examinations on both patients and fill out requisitions for chest films (to include the appropriate laterals).

Mr. Dean has rales anteriorly but his posterior base is clear. He has a white count of 11,000.

Miss Pulsifer is much more toxic, has rales and dullness to percussion posteriorly, and her white count is 18,000.

From your experience on the preceding page spreads, have you any roentgen evidence here for a hydropneumothorax in either patient? Why? Why not?

If you think pneumonic consolidation could explain either of the curious straight line interfaces, precisely what part of the lung would be involved? Anticipate the lateral film in each.

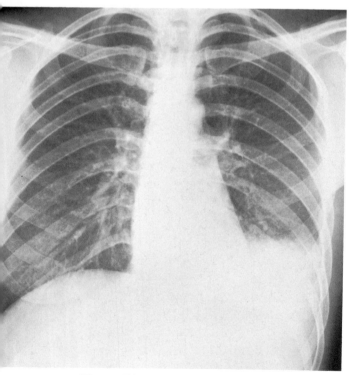

Figure 52   **ANN PULSIFER**

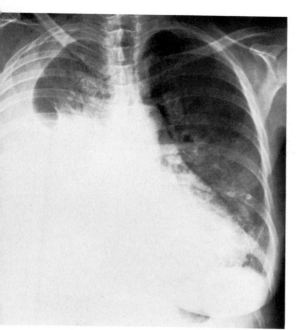

Figure 53   MRS. FOSTER

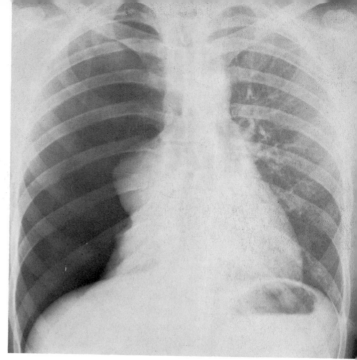

Figure 54   MR. ADAMS

Later you examine Mrs. Foster and Mr. Adams, who both come to the hospital because of **Increasing Dyspnea.**

Mrs. Foster is well known to the hospital and has had many admissions for cirrhosis associated with chronic alcoholism. She is not febrile.

Mr. Adams has not been seen here before and was well yesterday. He has had some chest pain for 24 hours but has no fever or cough.

What do you find in each on physical examination? Explain the dyspnea both dynamically and physiologically.

FOLD THE MARGIN OF THIS
PAGE IN TO THE CENTER OF
THE BOOK AND YOU WILL BE
ABLE TO EXAMINE THE
LATERAL FILMS ON MR. DEAN
AND MISS PULSIFER
TOGETHER WITH THEIR PA
CHEST FILMS. DO THE LATERAL
FILMS CHANGE YOUR MIND
ABOUT ANYTHING YOU HAD
DECIDED?

ANSWERS

Mr. Dean and Miss Pulsifer.
Neither of the "straight-line" interfaces could be a pleural fluid level.
There is nothing to indicate a hydropneumothorax since normal lung
markings are seen extending straight
to the chest wall. There is no curving
line in either patient to suggest pleural
fluid.

The lateral on Mr. Dean shows you
the triangular shadow across the heart
which you have come to associate with
middle lobe consolidation. The horizontal interface seen in the PA chest
film is consolidated between middle
lobe and aerated upper lobe. The heart/
lung interface in the PA view has been
preserved so Mr. Dean must have
pneumonia involving only the lateral
segment of his middle lobe, the medial
segment having been spared.

Miss Pulsifer's lost diaphragm is
explained when you see the lateral.
Only one diaphragmatic interface is
seen, the normal right. She has consolidation of the four basilar segments
of the left lower lobe and the apical
segment has been spared. The "straight
line" in the PA view is the irregular top
of the consolidation.

In Figures 57 and 58 you have
follow-up films on Miss Pulsifer. Note
the reappearance of *two* diaphragmatic
interfaces.

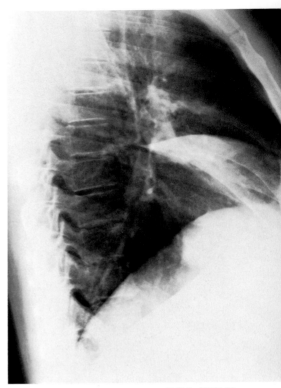

Figure 55   BILL DEAN

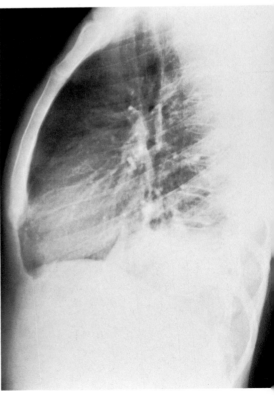

Figure 56   ANN PULSIFER

Mrs. Foster has a massive pleural effusion extending over the apex of the right lung and displacing the mediastinum to the left. Right thoracentesis showed clear fluid and 1500 cc. was removed. Dyspnea, mechanical in origin, was much relieved with the additional removal of two liters of abdominal ascitic fluid.

Mr. Adams has a pneumothorax with almost complete collapse of the right lung and slight shift of the mediastinum to the left, suggesting the possibility of tension pneumothorax. Of the four patients it would be Mr. Adams whom you should attend to first, of course, since tension pneumothorax can be a disaster and should be decompressed early. If you could have seen the chest fluoroscopy on this patient, how would his mediastinum have shifted with each inspiration and expiration? His dyspnea was appreciably relieved by prompt pleural decompression and re-expansion of the right lung. Dyspnea must have been the result of decreased oxygenation with only one working lung and great reduction in the venous return to the heart with such an increase in intrathoracic pressure.

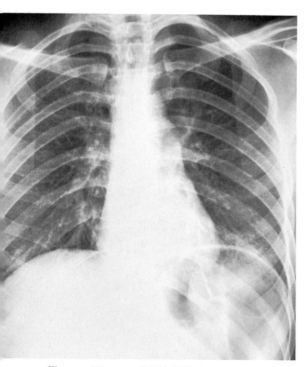

Figure 57   **ANN PULSIFER**

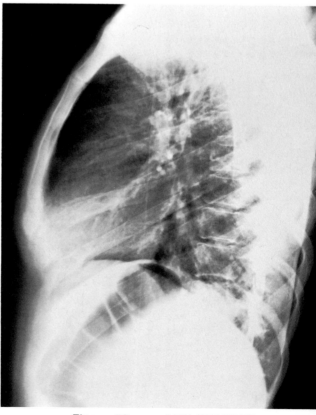

Figure 58   **ANN PULSIFER**

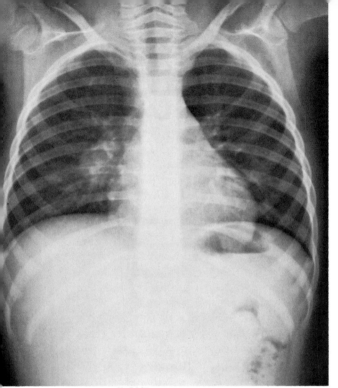

Figure 59   **A**

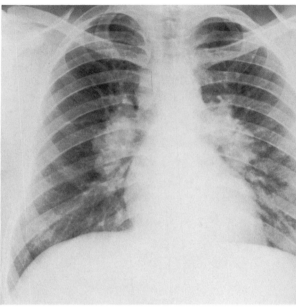

Figure 60   **B**

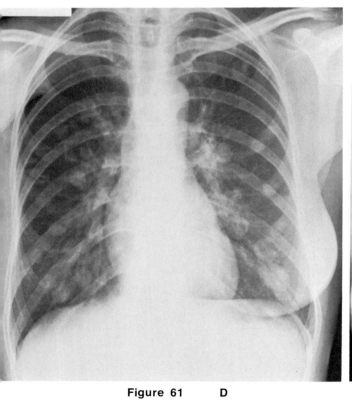

Figure 61   **D**

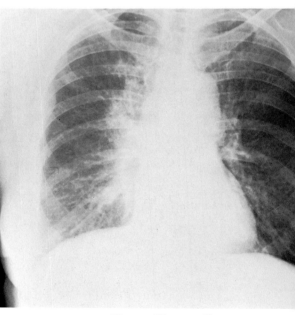

Figure 62   **E**

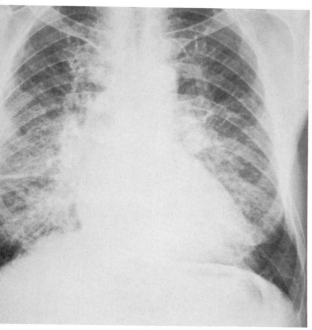

Figure 63   **C**

PROBLEMS

Are there any roentgen findings here which give you a clue as to the **Age** of any of these six patients?

On physical examination one of these patients had an **Enlarged Spleen** but is not acutely ill. Can you pick out which one?

Two patients have nontender **Cervical Lymph Nodes.** Which two?

Three are **Dyspneic.** Which three? Why are they short of breath?

Patient **F,** acutely ill with **Chest Pain,** has just been admitted to the emergency division. He claims he has never been sick a day in his life before this afternoon. Patient **C** has been sick in bed at home for two months. Both have **Enlarged Livers.** Why do you think they are enlarged and what would you expect to find on microscopic inspection of liver tissue?

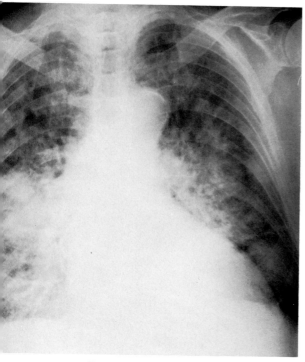

Figure 64   **F**

ANSWERS

Age — Patient **A** is a child; evident when you discover his unfused humeral epiphyses. Mr. **F** is an older man with a large heart and heavily calcified aorta.

The **Spleen** is visible and normal in the child, **A**. Patient **B** could have sarcoidosis or Hodgkin's disease. None of the other patients has findings suggesting any disease process usually associated with splenomegaly.

Both **A** and **B** had nontender **Cervical Nodes.** The child had glandular tuberculosis and a node in the right hilum which regressed under therapy. **B** had Hodgkin's disease (proved by node biopsy) and a big spleen. Figure 65 is his lateral film.

Patients **C** and **F** were **Dyspneic** because of cardiac failure, acute in **F** and chronic in **C**. (Note Kerley's B lines in Figure 63 in the right lower lung field near the chest wall and also the extrapleural edema.) Both these patients had been hypertensive for some time and have large hearts. Figure 68 shows Patient **C** a year earlier.

Patient **F** had a massive myocardial infarction a few hours ago and is in acute pulmonary edema.

Mr. **C** has big engorged hila and his **Large Liver** would show chronic passive congestion. With Patient **F**'s brief history his large liver was harder to explain until a week or so later (Fig. 69) when his edema had cleared on management and the pulmonary metastases from his unsuspected colon carcinoma emerged from their surrounding fluid. At autopsy a month later his liver was almost entirely replaced with carcinoma.

Patient **D** had a right mastectomy some time ago and now has many round pulmonary metastases. She was not dyspneic.

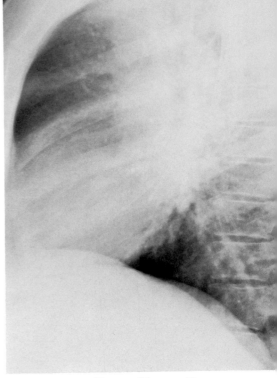

Figure 65   **B**

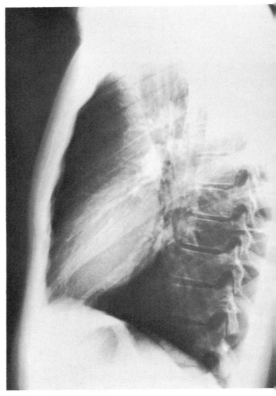

Figure 66   **NORMAL**

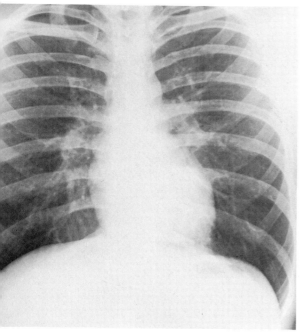

Figure 67   NORMAL

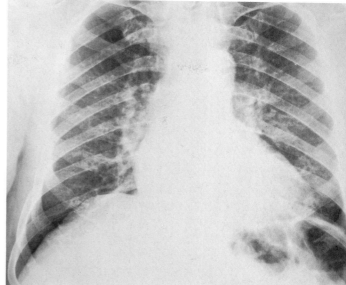

Figure 68   C

Patient **E** had a left mastectomy two years ago and now returns complaining of steadily increasing dyspnea. She has a widened mediastinal shadow and lymphangitic spread of carcinoma outward from the mediastinum into the peribronchial lymphatics. Mechanical pressure on her airway is responsible for her dyspnea.

Figure 67, a normal chest film, is supplied for comparison with all other hilar shadows.

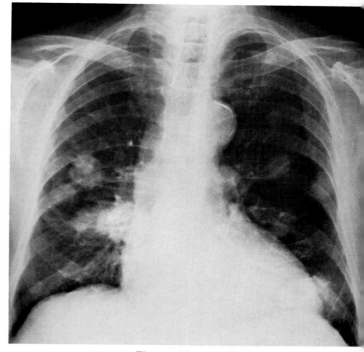

Figure 69   F

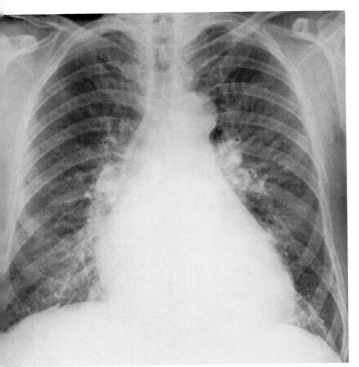

Figure 70   MR. A. DUPUY-BAMBLESCHNITZLER

FOUR PATIENTS WHO HAVE ALL BEEN EXPOSED TO TUBERCULOSIS . . .

Alexander Dupuy-Bambleschnitzler, 65, executive, finally complies enough with his wife's too frequently expressed concern for his health to submit to a physical check-up. He has been tired recently but blames it on the difficult labor situation at the plant. He has a cough, some dyspnea on exertion, and has not enjoyed his golf game recently because his feet are swollen and his shoes hurt. Past history is not helpful. The wife, who is present, informs you that two of his brothers had chronic cough and were believed by the family to have had tuberculosis. The patient is planning to drive to a sales meeting 500 miles away tonight. What is your procedure?

Tommy Payton, 9, has been sick with a cold at home for two days and is suddenly much worse. He is brought to your office by his mother because he coughed up a little bloody sputum. He has rales on the right, especially posteriorly, is coughing, flushed and breathes rapidly. Stat WBC is reported by your office nurse as 18,500, and she tells you his temperature is 102° F. He appears dehydrated. The mother, a social worker, tells you that a PPD done at school a week ago was negative. She says his grandmother, living with the family, had pulmonary tuberculosis years ago as a young woman. Decide on your differential diagnostic slate. How much does the film help? What will your management be?

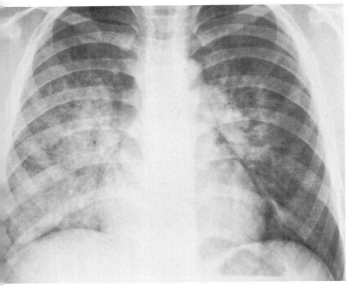

Figure 71   TOMMY PAYTON

Gordon Flashman, 28, printer's assistant, comes to you complaining of difficulty in breathing. He has lost 15 pounds in six months and is always tired. Except for chest findings apparent on this film, he has no other symptoms or signs and is afebrile. His hemogram is normal and he has no past medical history of any significance. His younger brother had been in a hospital with active tuberculosis but is now well. What are the diagnostic possibilities? How should you proceed?

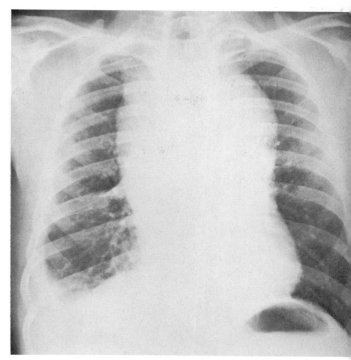

Figure 72   GORDON FLASHMAN

Antonio Spinelli, 58, consults you because of difficulty in breathing and a weight loss of 25 pounds in two months. He has what he describes as a cigarette cough but has not coughed up any sputum. His father died of tuberculosis 15 years ago after living with the patient the last two years of his life. Mr. Spinelli had a medical check-up four months ago, including a chest film, and was given a clean bill of health. When you examine him you find an inspiratory wheeze and his neck veins are dilated. What is the most probable among your diagnostic possibilities? How will you prove it?

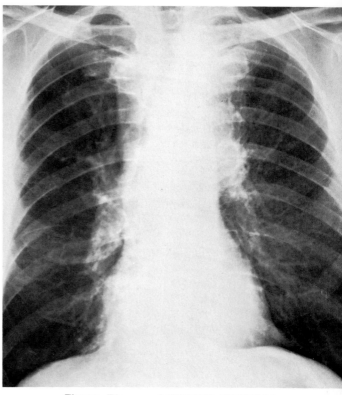

Figure 73   ANTONIO SPINELLI

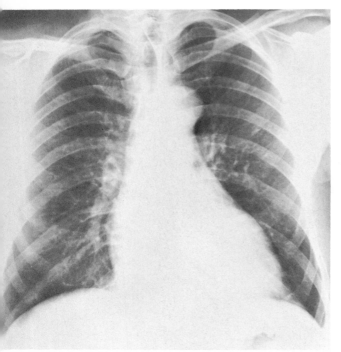

Figure 74   MR. D. B.

... BUT NONE OF WHOM HAD IT

Mr. Bambleschnitzler has a large heart, engorged hila, increased vascular pulmonary markings and Kerley's B lines. He is in early-to-moderate congestive failure. You persuade him to send his second-in-command (or Mrs. B.) to the sales meeting and admit him to the hospital. After two weeks on therapy he is much better. Figure 74 is his discharge film. (He has nothing to suggest pulmonary tuberculosis.)

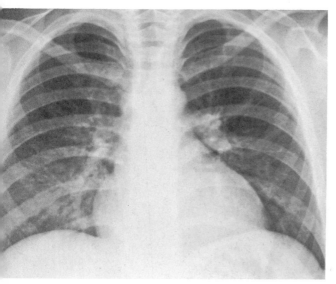

Figure 75   TOMMY P.

Tommy has a diffusely disseminated bronchopneumonia, more advanced on the right. Streptococci were obtained from his sputum. The film findings alone might just possibly be those of a fulminant pulmonary acid-fast infection in a child, but neither the very acute picture clinically nor the rapid recovery was consistent with tuberculosis. He recovered on antibiotics within a week. Figure 75 is his PA film at 48 hours. Figures 76 and 77 are his early and late lateral films.

(If you fold in the page margin you can look at all four films together.)

Mr. Flashman has a markedly widened mediastinal shadow and a right pleural effusion. The mass is confluent with the heart shadow and probably applied closely against it. The differential possibilities include all the anterior mediastinal masses which may be found in young adults. Of these, teratoma and lymphoma are the most likely in this patient. The possibility of tuberculosis, in spite of the history, is remote. Thoracentesis produced a clear, sterile fluid with no cells; it was probably, therefore, a mechanical transudate. Node biopsy showed lymphoma.

Mr. Spinelli's striking weight loss must be explained. His film shows a widened mediastinum and his physical findings suggest tracheal compression. (An overexposed film or a tomogram would have shown this better.) With this picture, the first consideration for a patient in his age group must be bronchogenic carcinoma with mediastinal metastases encasing the trachea and major bronchi. Often other structures are also involved, such as the superior vena cava, the esophagus, and the recurrent laryngeal or phrenic nerves. With a history of a normal chest film four months ago, his strikingly abnormal film findings are strong presumptive evidence for new growth rather than any sort of tuberculous involvement in spite of the history. Biopsy was taken of a supraclavicular node and radiation therapy started, but the patient died suddenly a week after this film was made. At autopsy he was found to have extensive early mediastinal spread from a dime-sized carcinoma in the right main stem bronchus. Bronchoscopic study had been unsatisfactory because of the tracheal narrowing to less than half its normal dimension.

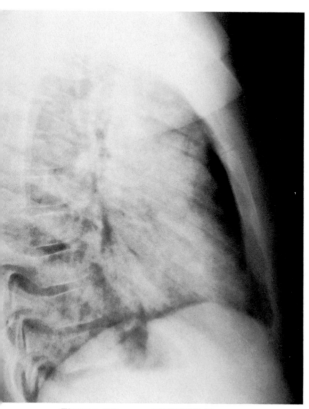

Figure 76   TOMMY P.

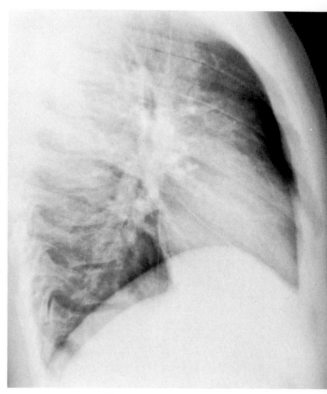

Figure 77   TOMMY P.

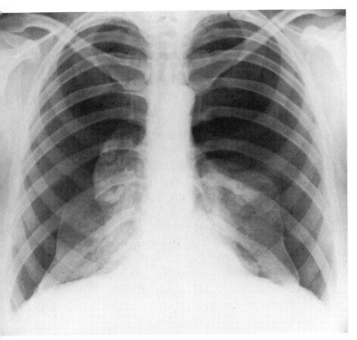

Figure 78   MRS. PARDIGGLE A

PROBLEM

Explain **Shortness of Breath** in each of these five patients. (Note that Figures 80 and 82 are of the same patient.) All were extremely ill; **C** and **E** had high fevers; the rest were afebrile.

Which have the bleakest prognoses?

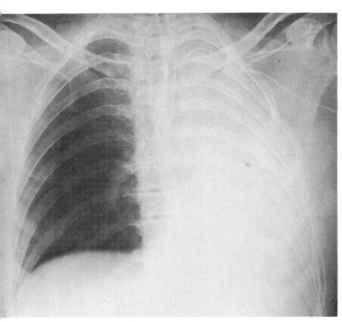

Figure 79   HAROLD SKIMPOLE B

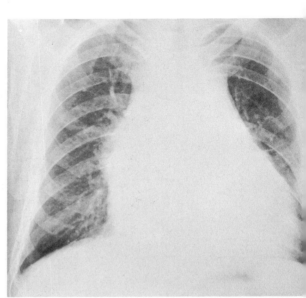

Figure 80   MR. SNAGSBY C

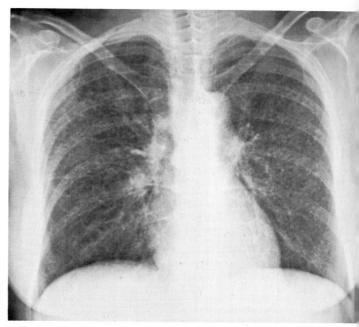

Figure 81   VOLUMNIA DEADLOCK D

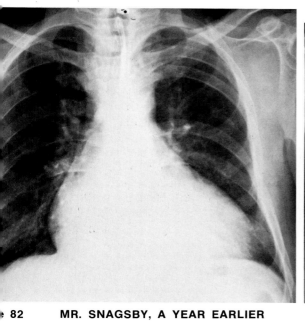

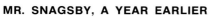

82   MR. SNAGSBY, A YEAR EARLIER

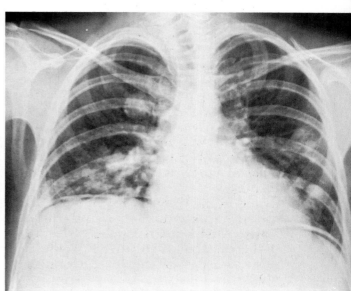

Figure 83   MR. TULKINGHAM E

ANSWERS

A, *Mrs. Pardiggle,* had sudden chest pain two hours ago while cleaning her basement and has been dyspneic at rest ever since. She has a bilateral 60 to 75 per cent pneumothorax. No lung markings are seen beyond the margins of the collapsing lungs. The white line bordering the lungs is visceral pleura seen tangentially. Note how the heart/lung interfaces are disappearing as the roentgen density of the lung approaches that of heart muscle. Mrs. Pardiggle had had two previous episodes of spontaneous pneumothorax; she probably ruptured emphysematous blebs during her housecleaning exertions. Her dyspnea was, of course, the result of sudden decrease in functioning lung tissue and was present even as she lay quietly in bed.

This is an example of collapse of lung due to compression from air in the pleural space.

B, *Mr. Skimpole,* has a collapsed left lung but no pneumothorax to push it in against the mediastinum. This is a straight sagittal film and, therefore, there is a valid and marked displacement of the mediastinum to the left. The density occupying the left hemithorax is, then, the heart and great vessels, together with the airless left lung lying against the chest wall. Dyspnea is due to sudden decrease in functioning lung tissue.

Now note that the endotracheal tube is in the *right* main bronchus. The film was made because the patient, postoperative after an emergency appendectomy with general anesthesia, rapidly became cyanotic and tachypneic in the recovery room. When the catheter was withdrawn well above the carina and suction applied, the left lung re-expanded quite readily. (Figure 84 was made two hours after Figure 79.)

Here collapse is of a quite different character and the airlessness of the lung is due to bronchial obstruction and secondary resorption of air.

C, *Mr. Snagsby,* with his marked cardiomegaly and missing left sixth rib, at once suggests a patient who has had heart valve surgery. However, his surgery (to a stenosed aortic valve) was carried out two years ago. Figure 82 is a film made a short time ago before his present illness. Note the difference in the width of the mediastinum. He was admitted with substernal pain and a temperature of 105° F. He was delirious and extremely restless. Surgical decompression of the mediastinum revealed a large mediastinal abscess. This was drained and the patient put on high doses of antibiotics. After a stormy period of recovery an additional complaint of dysphagia could be investigated by barium swallow, and an esophageal carcinoma was found which had perforated into the mediastinum. His dyspnea was due to mechanical compression of the trachea and bronchi from edema and exudate under pressure.

D, *Mrs. Deadlock,* had an occupational history of having worked (for six months only and that 20 years ago) in a tubular illumination plant making fluorescent light bulbs. Her dyspnea has been gradually increasing and her chest film shows the myriads of small disseminated shadows throughout both lungs which are seen in injury to the lung from beryllium. These represent the shadows of granulomas and scar tissue, and they are less striking on the chest film than microscopically because of the "subtraction effect" of the marked accompanying emphysema which is present. The dyspnea is explained by the extensive parenchymal changes and associated thickening of the alveolar walls which cause "alveolar-capillary block" and interference with the exchange of gases.

E, *Mr. Tulkingham,* has high diaphragms with air under both and multiple round densities in the lungs. He had a bilateral adrenal ablation a year ago for adrenal carcinoma and has been on maintenance hormone management. This was directly related to the perforation of his gastric ulcer four days ago. At the time this film was made he had peritonitis and high, fixed diaphragms. His dyspnea was due to pain, limited diaphragmatic motion and small tidal air.

The curious names? All characters in Dickens' Bleak House. *C,* **D,** *and* **E** *had very bleak prognoses, but* **A** *and* **B** *recovered promptly.*

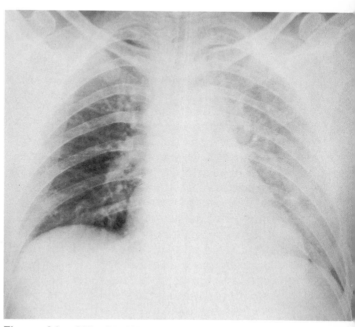

Figure 84   MR. SKIMPOLE—LATER THE SAME NIGHT.

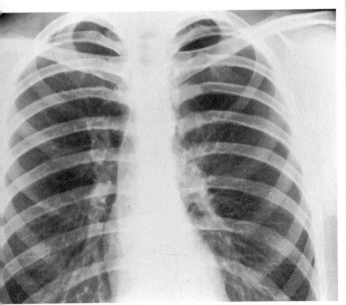

Figure 85　　A

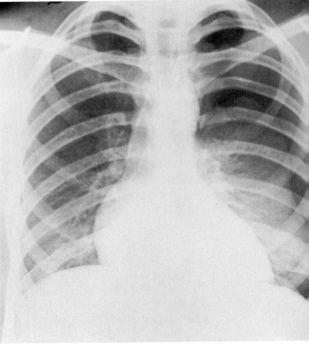

Figure 86　　B

PROBLEMS

Patient **A** had slight chest pain an hour ago. Study the film, comparing carefully the markings in bilaterally symmetrical interspaces.

Now perhaps you have recognized the margin of partially collapsed left lung and the presence of pneumothorax on that side. The air imprisoned in the pleural space is a trifle more radiolucent than blood-perfused lung even at inspiration. At expiration this "cushion of air" is compressed.

Now study **B,** an expiration film made on the same patient. There the difference in density between pneumothorax and partially collapsed left lung is much greater, and there is a striking contrast between the density of the two lungs, something which was not evident at once even on the original film for **A.** The implication is clear – we know that both lungs are less radiolucent at expiration than when fully expanded, and here in **B** one is contrasting *three* different densities: normal right lung at expiration, partially collapsed left lung also at expiration, and free air in the pleural space. The *difference* between the latter two is greater at expiration than it is at inspiration, and the expiration film is therefore much more likely to show the presence of a small pneumothorax which might otherwise escape our notice. Perhaps it would be well to order such a series routinely in patients with sudden chest pain.

Note, too, the short horizontal fluid/air interface in the left costophrenic sinus, another clue to the presence of pneumothorax. The mediastinum appears to bow to the right on both films. Now study **C-D** and **E-F,** two more pairs of inspiration-expiration films. Both patients had had chest pain of two hours' duration, but were perfectly well that morning. (Be sure to decide about mediastinal shift.)

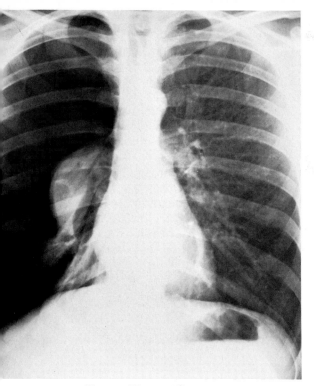

Figure 87   **C**

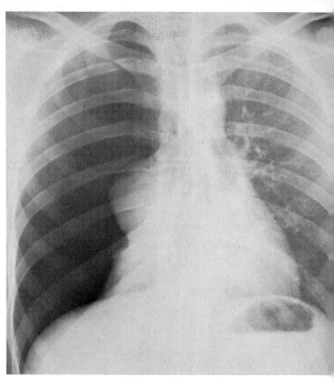

Figure 88   **D**

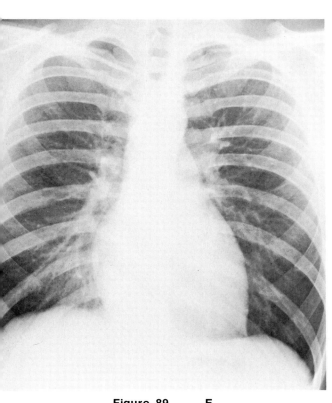

Figure 89   **E**

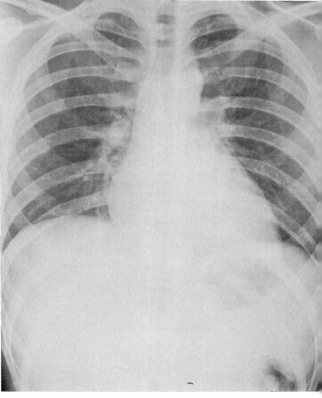

Figure 90   **F**

ANSWERS

C-D has a large right pneumothorax and almost total collapse of the right lung with rather pronounced mediastinal shift to the left on expiration. The picture raises the question of a tension pneumothorax. Note how the trapped pleural air seems to bulge into the left hemithorax across the heart shadow in **D.** At surgical decompression there was a dramatic release of air.

E-F is a normal chest film at inspiration and expiration. The patient was apparently having an acute gallbladder attack and possibly passing a stone. He subsequently localized his pain to the upper abdomen and back and was transiently jaundiced. **F** was made first, rejected because of the poor inspiration, and then **E** was obtained.

If you called **E** a normal chest film, be sure to recognize with relief and encouragement your own progress in discrimination and judgment about roentgen findings. Remember, it is always a normal chest film until you can find something definitely wrong with it.

The films on this page spread were *all* made on patients with **Chest Pain of a Few Hours' Duration,** so you have another chance to differentiate between valid roentgen findings and others that must be discounted for one reason or another. All these patients were in the hospital for at least one night.

(Study in **lettered** order. Answers on Page 47.)

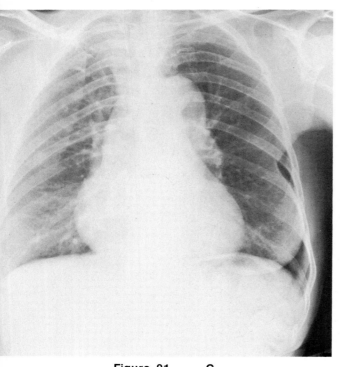

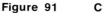

Figure 91   **C**

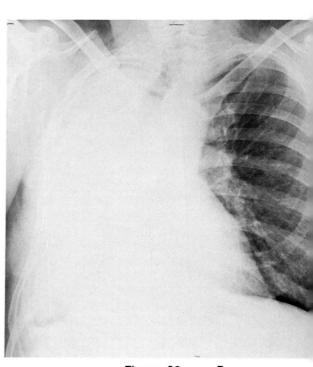

Figure 92   **D**

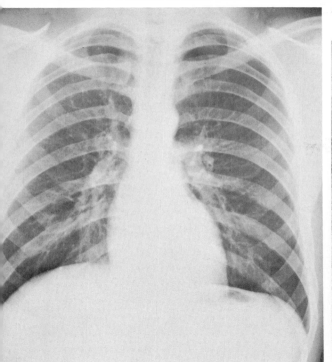

Figure 93   A

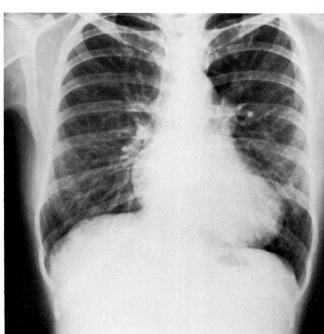

Figure 94   B

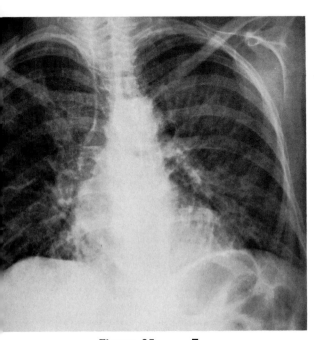

Figure 95   E

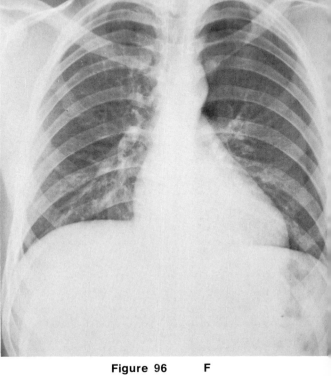

Figure 96   F

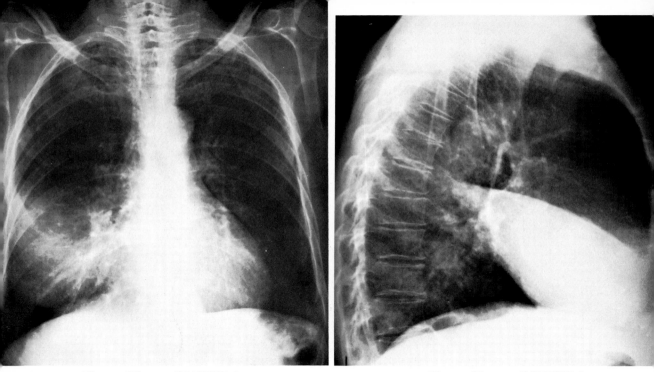

Figure 97   PATIENT L

Figure 98   PATIENT L

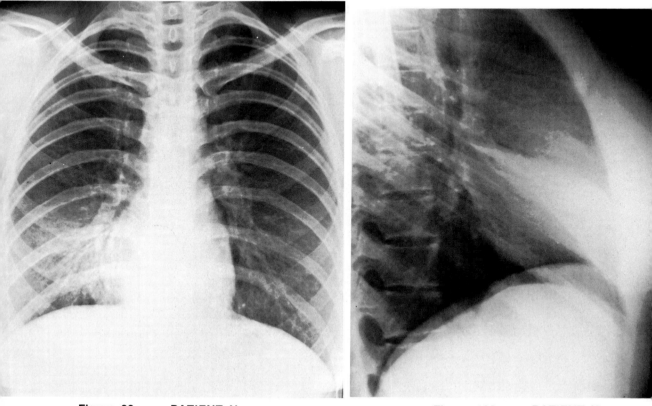

Figure 99   PATIENT N

Figure 100   PATIENT N

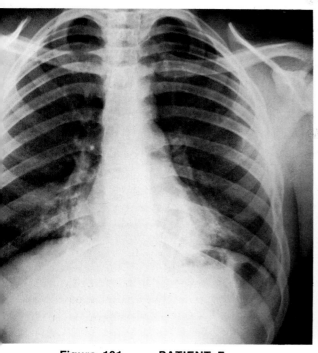

Figure 101   PATIENT F

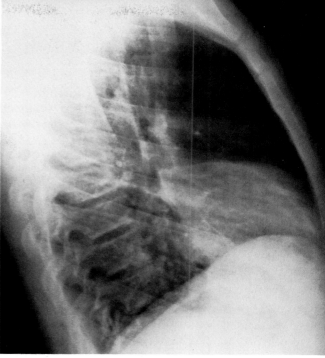

Figure 102   PATIENT F

REVIEW OF LOBAR CONSOLIDATION, COLLAPSE AND MEDIASTINAL SHIFT

Fill in the appropriate patient's initial. If none fits, enter a zero.

IN THIS GROUP,
ONLY PATIENT _____ HAS SHIFT OF THE ENTIRE MEDIASTINUM TO ONE SIDE.

ONLY THE R. _____ L. IS INVOLVED IN PATIENT L.

IN PATIENT _____ THE LOWER PART OF THE MEDIASTINUM ONLY IS SHIFTED.

THERE IS R.U.L.
ATELECTASIS IN _____

ONLY PATIENT _____ HAS MORE THAN ONE LOBE INVOLVED.

PATIENT _____ HAS ONE WHOLE LUNG COLLAPSED.

IN PATIENT _____ ONE POSTERIOR DIAPHRAGMATIC INTERFACE IS LOST.

PATIENT _____ PROBABLY HAS PNEUMONIA WITHOUT ANY ATELECTASIS.

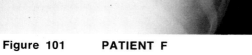

Figure 103   PATIENT I

ANSWERS TO PROBLEMS ON PAGES 44 AND 45

If your filled-in answers are correct, you have a vertical acrostic reading "I'M NO FOOL." Congratulations on both counts!

Patient **L** has a R.M.L. consolidation with no decrease in size of the lobe (lateral view). The right heart/lung interface has been lost. The mediastinum is not shifted. In the PA view you are seeing the vessels for the lower lobe superimposed on homogeneously dense middle lobe.

Patient **N** had a R.M.L. pneumonia clinically, too, but her middle lobe is markedly decreased in size as seen in the lateral view. There is much too much right heart and too little left heart shadow in the PA view, indicating a swing of the lower part of the mediastinum to the right. The trachea is in its normal position. The right heart border is quite often still visible in the PA view in R.M.L. atelectasis because there is not enough airless lung lying against the heart to obscure it.

Patient **F** has densities on both sides of the heart, smudging its right and left borders and indicating lung density in both the right middle lobe and the lingula of the left upper lobe. There may also be some patchy involvement in the lower lobes, but it does not coalesce enough to obscure the diaphragm posteriorly.

Patient **I** has partial collapse of the left upper lobe which has obscured the left heart border and shifted the mediastinum sharply to the left. The whole left lung *could not* be atelectatic because the left leaf of the diaphragm is so clearly seen. This must mean the left *lower* lobe is well aerated. This patient had an obstructing carcinoma of the left upper lobe bronchus. There was also a mass of nodes at the left hilum, seen vaguely outlined here by air in the lower lobe.

Nobody has a right upper lobe collapse.

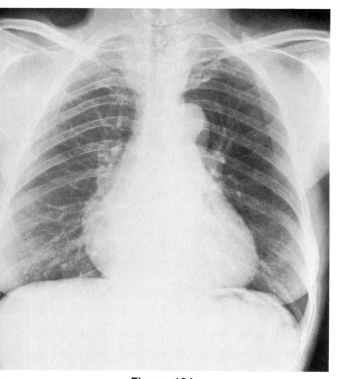

Figure 104

ANSWERS TO PROBLEMS ON PAGES 42 AND 43

C shows a fair degree of rotation, but *is* the heart really enlarged? Figure 104 is a film made on the same patient with a straight sagittal beam. Tip the margins so that Figures 91 and 104 can be examined side by side. Chest pain in this patient proved to be due to angina. She was hypertensive and the heart is larger than normal.

There is also slight rotation in Figure 95, but Mr. **E** was very ill, very dyspneic, very anxious, and in a good deal of pain. He was in acute left heart failure, the result of a myocardial infarction of several hours' duration. He was very hard to position, and you have definite roentgen signs here and need not repeat the film.

There is no rotation in young Mr. **A,** whose film probably appears normal. His rather small, spontaneous pneumothorax on the left could be seen in retrospect on the original film but had been missed until an expiration film (**F**) was made. You can now see the lateral margin of left lung about 25 per cent collapsed. The upper mediastinum is not shifted, although the heart tilts to the left on expiration. Recovery was prompt.

Patient **B,** with no rotation and diaphragms fairly well down, has exaggerated and somewhat tortuous vascular markings throughout both lungs (compare the same parts of each lung with **A** beside it). The cardiac shadow is generous and shows left ventricular preponderance. The patient had the characteristic murmur of interatrial septal defect, later confirmed by angiocardiogram. The suspiciously nodular hilar shadows in patients with shunt are exemplified here and produced by dilated and tortuous pulmonary veins and arteries. The size of the left ventricle in this patient was due to increased work necessary to carry an overload of the lesser circulation of 30 per cent return to the right atrium through the shunt. Chest pain in this patient, however, was esophageal and due to a poorly chewed piece of meat lodged near the cardia. The pain was relieved when it passed through into the stomach.

The patient shown in **D** must have either a collapsed or an absent right lung. The left diaphragm is below the tenth rib and the clavicles are symmetrical in appearance; therefore, the strikingly shifted position of the trachea must be a valid finding. If you knew this patient's chest film had been normal a few months ago, lung collapse should be your first thought, provided the patient does not have a pneumonectomy scar (this one did).

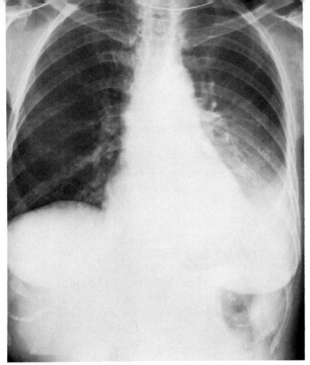

Figure 105   A

PROBLEMS

At the left you have two patients with fever whose PA chest films show left lower lung field densities of some kind. A systematic analysis of the PA films alone should inform you (1) what part of the lung is involved, and (2) how the related left laterals would differ from each other.

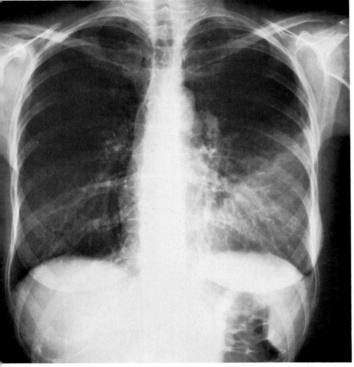

Figure 106   B

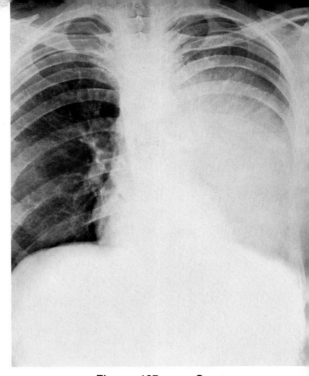

Figure 107   **C**

PROBLEMS

Here you have two more patients with trouble on the left side. Analyze their PA views with regard to degree of inspiration, rotation if any, mediastinal shift if any, and lobe involved. Predict the related left lateral chest films.

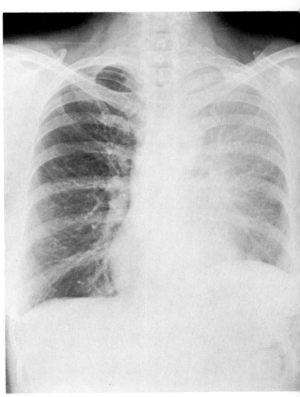

Figure 108   **D**

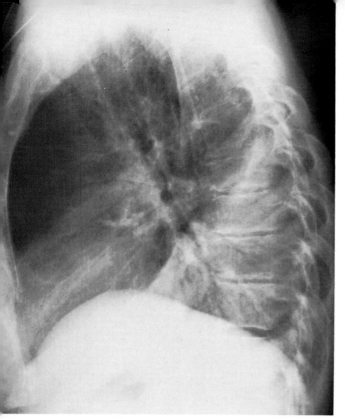

Figure 109   A

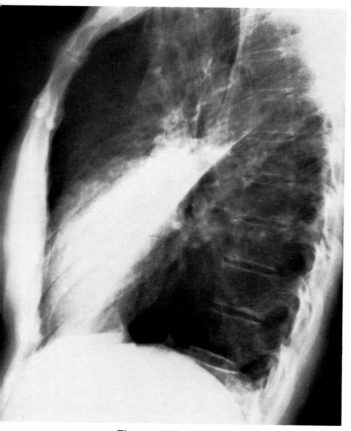

Figure 110   B

ANSWERS TO PAGE 48

Mrs. **A** has a lower lung field density which obscures the diaphragm but not the heart border.

The dark shadow of the left lower lobe bronchus is *also* seen to extend downward across the heart border, suggesting that it may have consolidated lung tissue surrounding it (an air bronchogram). There are, therefore, three roentgen findings on this single film to suggest left *lower* lobe consolidation: lost diaphragmatic interface, heart/lung interface preserved, and an air bronchogram involving the lower lobe bronchus.

The left lateral film (Fig. 109) shows a wedge of density overlying the lower thoracic vertebrae bounded anteriorly by the slanting major fissure and only one visible diaphragm (the normal right). Note the air bronchogram, but do not be confused by the fact that you are *also* seeing white branching trunks; these represent the normal vascular supply to the *right* lower lobe surrounded by air!

Mrs. **B** has a lung density which obscures the heart border but not the diaphragm, roentgen findings which should at once suggest to you consolidation of the anterior part of the lung lying against the heart (*i.e.*, the lingular division of the left upper lobe). The related lateral (Fig. 110) shows the anticipated white wedge overlying the heart shadow.

Be sure to study the two problem PA films matched against the two laterals by placing the margin of page 50 in the middle of page 48.

ANSWERS TO PAGE 49

(Now place the margin of page 49 in the center seam.)

Patient **C** has left lower lobe consolidation in spite of the presence of clear interface boundaries for both heart and diaphragm. This may often be so when there is some atelectasis of the lower lobe so that the major fissure is displaced posteriorly and the lingula somewhat overexpanded. In Patient **A** the PA view was made leaning farther forward. In Patient **C** there is a marked degree of kyphosis present so that the lower lobe "lives" farther back in the chest. Remember then that the heart border is a more dependable index than the diaphragm in the PA view in questions of lower lobe involvement and that the disappearance of the posterior segment of left diaphragm in the lateral clinches the matter in patients like Mrs. **C.** (She also has a hiatus hernia, by the way, with a fluid level above the diaphragm.)

Patient **D** has a high left diaphragm, clearly seen, and her left heart border is obscured. This should immediately suggest collapse of the left upper lobe, and the lateral film (Fig. 112) confirms that interpretation of the findings (the crescentic wedge of density against the sternum overlying part of the heart shadow). Its sharp posterior border indicates the position of the major fissure and the anterior margin of the overexpanded left lower lobe. Note two diaphragmatic shadows and the normal spine density compared with Figure 111.

Patients **A, B,** and **C** had pneumonia clinically and recovered. Patient **D** had an obstructing carcinoma of the left upper lobe bronchus with 75 per cent collapse of that lobe.

(Be sure to study the differences between the four laterals on pages 50 and 51 together.)

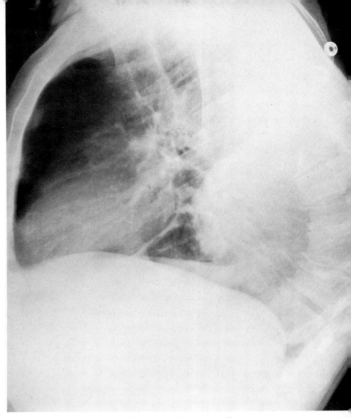

Figure 111   **C**

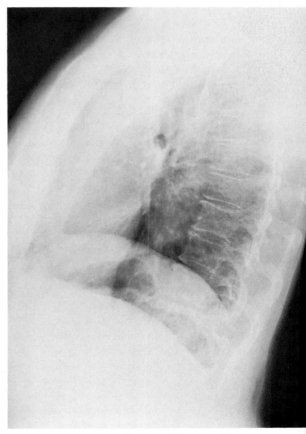

Figure 112   **D**

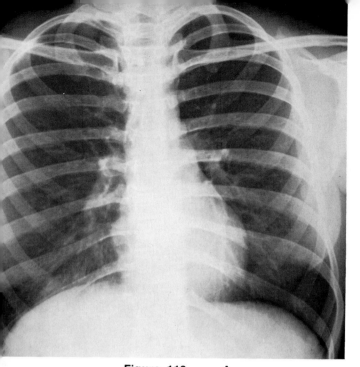

Figure 113   **A**

PROBLEM

Five particularly desirable prospective technical employees for your hospital come up for review medically, and you have to decide whether they should be hired.

A, B, D, and **E** have positive skin tests with medium strength PPD. **C** is negative but has some nontender cervical nodes and you think you can feel his spleen. He is coughing but afebrile. **A** and **E** have slight elevations of temperature and **E** also coughs, although he is obviously a chain smoker.

Here are their chest films. (The radiologist's reports have been withheld and you are on your own.) Examine their films, interspace for interspace, using any other films in the book as norm controls, and decide what you would recommend. Remember that good technicians are hard to find and each of these five people is badly wanted by one of your laboratories, no equally well-trained applicants being available.

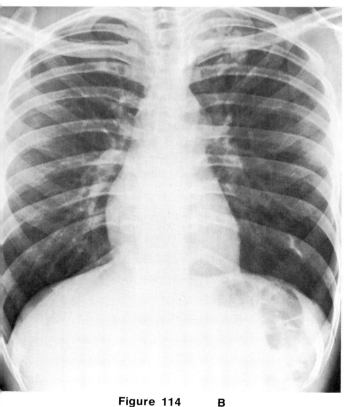

Figure 114   **B**

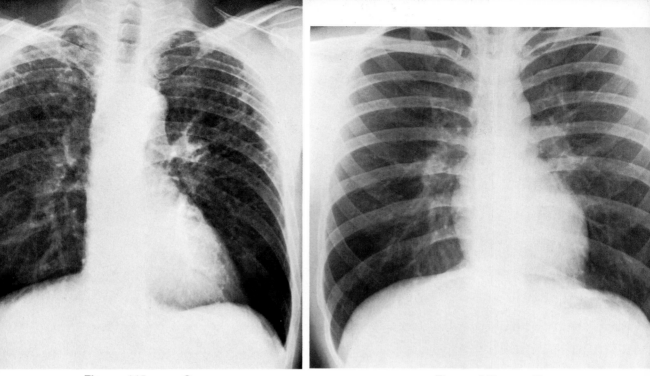

Figure 115   C

Figure 116   D

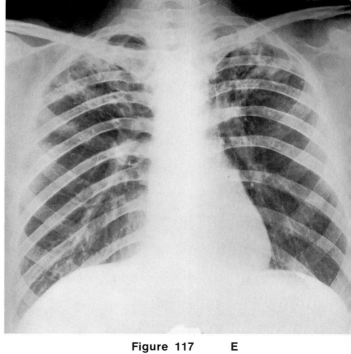

Figure 117   E

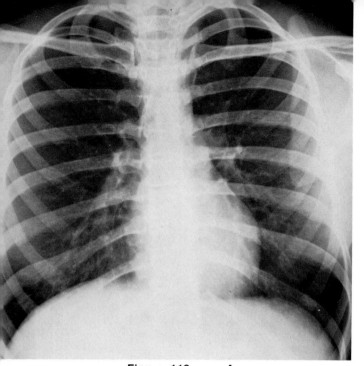

Figure 118   A

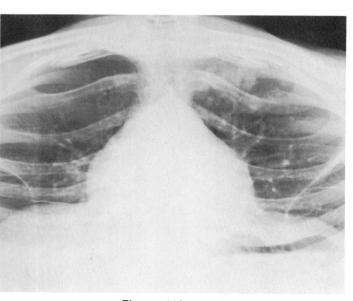

Figure 119   B

ANSWERS

Applicant **A** has a patch of density in the ninth interspace close to the right diaphragm. There is nothing like it in the corresponding interspace on the left. The rest of this young lady's chest film is normal. On further questioning she said she had not been feeling very well for a week before the film was made. This is a very unlikely location for acid-fast involvement (not impossible — just very improbable). Figure 118 shows you her check film. In the interval of 12 days the patch has almost completely cleared. This patient was judged to have had a minor unrecognized bronchopneumonia clearing without treatment and was hired.

Applicant **B** is another story. In the classic upper lobe location for tuberculosis this patient has a soft, cloudy density on the left. An apical lordotic film (Fig. 119) confirms its presence. This patient should probably not be employed anywhere for a few weeks while the lesion is being treated.

Applicant **C** with his nontender nodes, questionable spleen, negative skin test, and persistent cough without fever does not suggest tuberculosis clinically. His chest film shows a fine linear infiltration throughout both lung fields, rather diffuse and uniform in distribution. The hila are in normal position and seem rather thickened though not definitely nodular. Biopsy of a node confirmed the clinical suspicion of sarcoidosis. The patient was placed on therapy and employed. He made an excellent recovery and a chest film two years later appeared entirely normal.

Applicant **D** has a normal chest film. He was in excellent health and, like you and me, has a positive tuberculin skin test at age 20 without ever having had the disease. His health has remaining good and now, three years later, he is the valued senior technician in his laboratory.

Applicant **E** has bilateral infiltrative densities also in the upper lobes. In addition there are round, white-margined radiolucent areas on both sides which suggest cavities. Note, too, that the vascular trunks to the lower lobes have an appearance suggesting that they are stretched, and the hila seem high in relation to the heart shadow. This generally implies a very considerable decrease in size of the upper lobes, retraction from scarring rather than atelectasis. The upper lobes are probably, therefore, much more involved than they appear to be on first inspection. Although tuberculosis is never actually a roentgen diagnosis but rather a bacteriologic one, here the radiologist will undoubtedly inform you (perhaps in the way he phrases his report) that there is a 99 per cent probability that you will find this patient has bilateral active upper lobe tuberculosis and a positive sputum. With his degree of scarring his chances for ultimate cure are probably not good enough to warrant his employment.

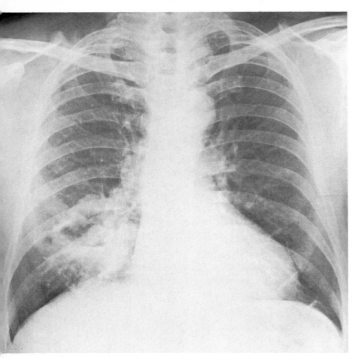

Figure 120   **JOHN C.**

PROBLEMS

You have five patients with productive cough and bloody sputum. The three women are febrile; the men are not.

Study their films carefully and then check out the **Roentgen Findings** listed below, entering the initial of the patient's surname in the appropriate blank. If the finding is not present on any film, enter a zero.

_____ HAS A THIN-WALLED CAVITY *AND* A CALCIFIED PRIMARY COMPLEX.

_____ SHOWS A SIGNIFICANT DEGREE OF ROTATION.

_____ = THE NUMBER OF PATIENTS IN THIS GROUP WHOSE ACTIVE LESION *MUST* BE IN THE UPPER LOBE.

_____ HAS A STRAIGHT LINE WHICH COULD BE EITHER A FLUID LEVEL WITHIN A LARGE LOWER LOBE CAVITY *OR* THE MINOR FISSURE WITH SOLID LUNG BENEATH IT IN MIDDLE LOBE.

_____ HAS MEDIASTINAL SHIFT.

_____ HAS A MASS DENSITY WHICH COULD NOT BE ENTIRELY IN THE RIGHT MIDDLE LOBE.

_____ = THE NUMBER OF CAVITIES IN FIGURE 124.

_____ HAS A THIN-WALLED CAVITY AND FLUID LEVEL BEHIND THE LEFT VENTRICLE AGAINST THE DIAPHRAGM.

_____ HAS A LUCENT AREA SUGGESTING A CAVITY IN THE LEFT UPPER LOBE.

_____ HAS A CAVITY WITH AN IRREGULAR WALL SUGGESTING BROKEN-DOWN TUMOR.

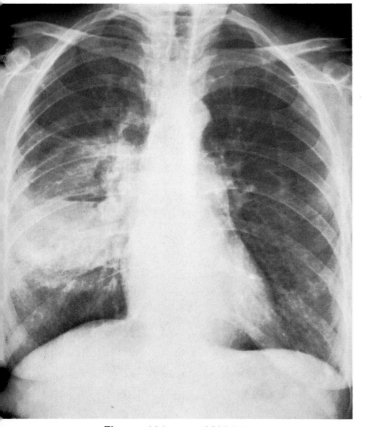

Figure 121   **AMANDA T.**

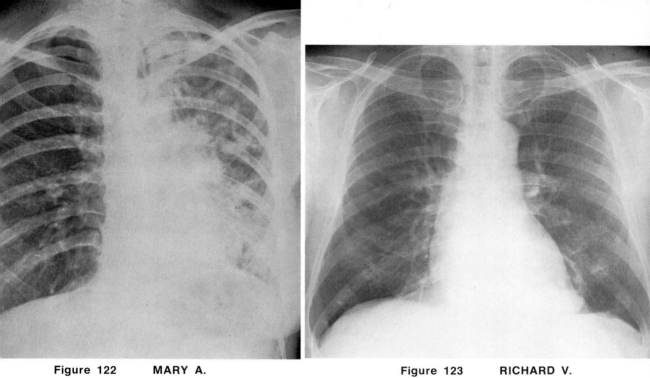

Figure 122   MARY A.

Figure 123   RICHARD V.

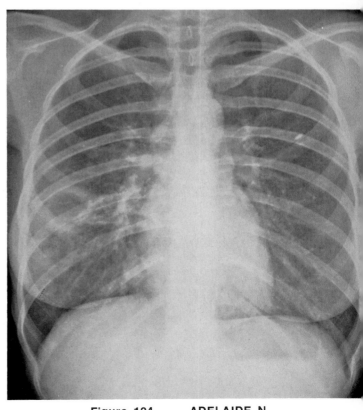

Figure 124   ADELAIDE N.

ANSWERS

If you have made all the right decisions, you have a vertical acrostic which spells "cavitation" . . . upside down.

John C. is a man in his sixties, as suggested by the prominent unrolled aorta and left ventricle. He was afebrile but coughing up a copious bloody sputum. His film shows a broken-down lesion, probably in the right lower lobe. The wall of the abscess is irregular in thickness and there are rounded masses projecting into the central cavity. At surgery a necrotic excavated carcinoma was found.

Amanda T., admitted with fever and bloody sputum, has some sort of straight line interface extending out from her right hilum. This might be the minor fissure with consolidated right middle lobe below it. However, the density in her right lung extends upward too far to *limit* it to the middle lobe. There are two possible explanations: either she has two separate areas of consolidation (one in the middle lobe and one behind it in the apex of the lower lobe) *or* the straight line represents a fluid level in a large abscess in the apex of the lower lobe and the middle lobe is clear. The lateral film (Fig. 125) gives you the answer.

Mary A., with fever and blood-streaked sputum, clearly has left upper lobe involvement with a cavity in the fourth interspace just below the mid clavicle. The left upper lobe must be involved because the trachea is shifted to the left (there is no rotation). The sputum was positive and the patient never responded well to therapy. Figure 127 is her chest film a year later, with the left lower lobe now also involved. Figure 128 is a specimen radiograph of her inflated lungs at necropsy with the arterial supply injected with opaque.

Richard V. has a normal chest film except for the fluid level behind the heart. Figure 126 is his lateral film. Any fluid- and air-filled structure near the midline and especially near the diaphragm brings the esophagus into question. A swallow of barium proved this to be a hiatus hernia. Mr. V.'s cough and sputum were later shown to relate to bronchiectasis, seldom visible on plain chest films like these.

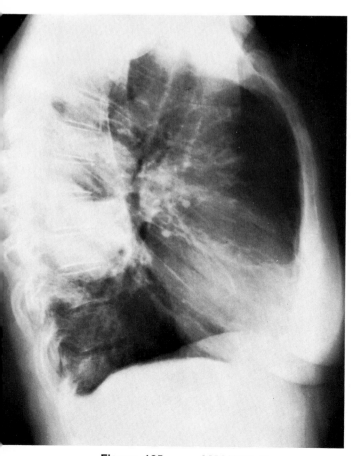

Figure 125   AMANDA T.

Adelaide N. has a soft, thin-walled abscess cavity in her right lung and a calcified primary complex in her left, overlying the sixth rib. The location of the cavity (lower part of upper lobe or in lower lobe) is an unusual one for tuberculosis in a patient with clear upper lobes. From its roentgen appearance this could just as well be a nonspecific lung abscess, but the mediastinal shadow is slightly widened and the hila suggest nodular thickening. The sputum was found to be loaded with acid-fast bacilli.

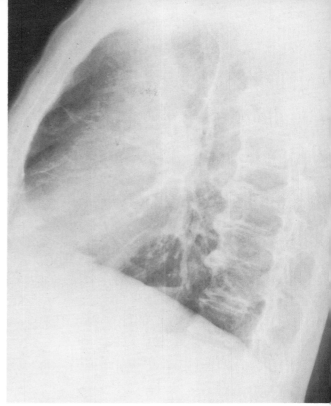

Figure 126   RICHARD V.

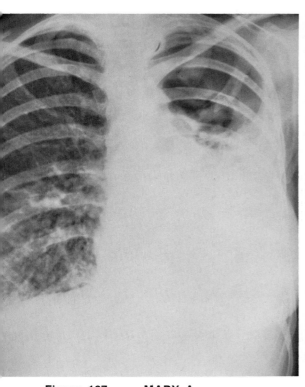

Figure 127   MARY A.

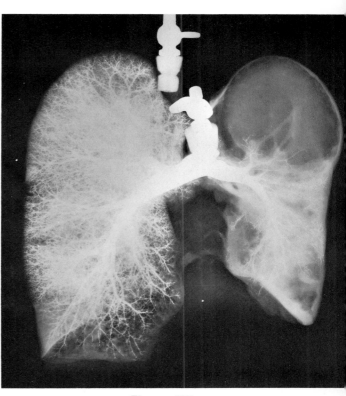

Figure 128

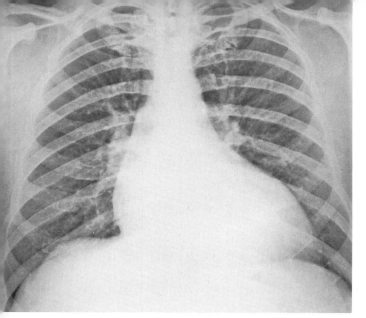

Figure 129   MR. ALEXANDER AGE 35

FOUR PATIENTS PRESENTING WITH CNS SYMPTOMS

Mr. Alexander, an accountant, consults you because of fainting spells, sometimes preceded by dizziness. Twice in the past six months he has been found unconscious and convulsing at the top of the subway stairs on his way home from work. He had rheumatic fever at age 16 and knows he has had a murmur ever since.

Mr. Baldwin, a linotype operator, has had no medical attention of any kind for years and has no past medical history of interest. He comes to clinic now because of several episodes of pulsatile headache produced by exercise. The headache always disappears after rest, but he then develops numbness and a pins-and-needles sensation in his right hand and in the right side of his mouth. The mouth twitches and he sometimes has trouble finding words.

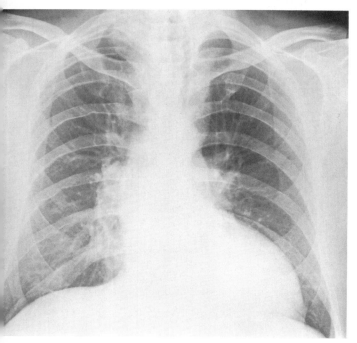

Figure 130   MR. BALDWIN AGE 55

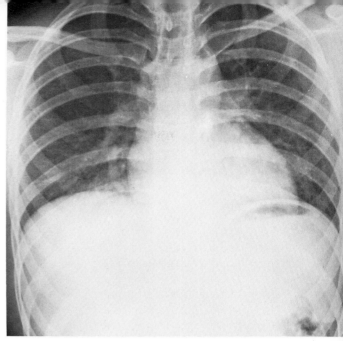

Figure 131   MR. PERKINS AGE 25

Mr. Perkins, a truckdriver, says he has been a heavy drinker since age 17. His girl will not marry him unless he stops drinking. Several times in the past three months he has stopped, and each time he has had several grand mal seizures within 24 hours, relieved when he began drinking again.

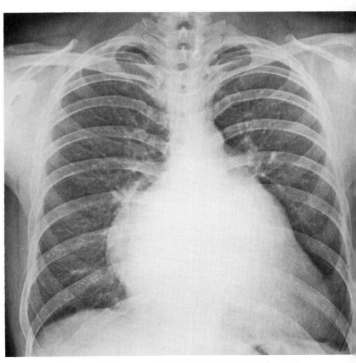

Figure 132   MR. BROMSON AGE 35

Mr. Bromson, a bookie, says he had an episode of profound dizziness with nausea and vomiting one month ago which gradually cleared over a period of several days during which everything "started spinning" whenever he turned his head to the right. A week ago on his way home from the track he fainted at the wheel of his car and had an automobile accident caused by his running into Mr. Perkins' truck, which was passing on his left.

ANSWERS

(Place margin of Page 62 in the middle of Page 60.)

Aortic Stenosis with Stokes-Adams Syndrome

Mr. Alexander had a loud systolic murmur heard best in the second right interspace and transmitted into the neck. Neurologic examination was normal. A diagnosis of effort-initiated Stokes-Adams syncopal attacks was made due to insufficient perfusion of the brainstem and vestibular nuclei in periods of prolonged asystole. The film shows left ventricular preponderance, a small aorta and engorged hila. Even in the absence of rib-notching, the whole picture might have been consistent with coarctation of the aorta rather than aortic stenosis except that the blood pressures were entirely within normal limits and uniform, with good femoral pulses. The auscultatory findings and his history of rheumatic fever make clear a diagnosis of pure rheumatic aortic stenosis with ventricular hypertrophy and Stokes-Adams episodes.

High Coarctation of the Aorta; Ischemia of Left Cerebrum

Mr. Baldwin had a BP of 170/100 in the right arm but much lower pressures in the left arm and both legs. Femoral pulses were very faint but present, presumably because of the very extensive collateral circulation which was evident with pulsating vessels around the right scapula. The coarctation must be high and involve the ostium of the left carotid in view of the findings and the story, which implies ischemia of the left parietal and frontal lobes (tingling and expressive aphasia). Note the notching of ribs predominantly on the right. The patient died a month later at home from a cerebral hemorrhage.

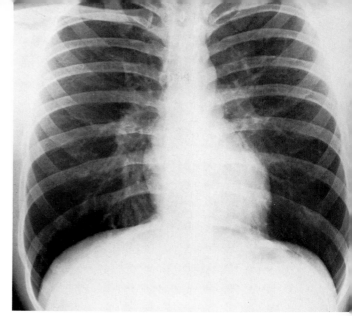

Figure 133

(Now place the margin of page 61 in the center seam between pages 62 and 63.)

Normal Chest Film at Expiration; "Rum Fits"

Mr. Perkins has been having seizures in response to withdrawal of alcohol. Except for a poor inspiration, his chest film is normal. (Figure 133 is his inspiration film.)

Rheumatic Heart Disease with Emboli to the Brain

Mr. Bromson obviously has advanced rheumatic heart disease with a greatly dilated left atrium and hypertrophied left ventricle. His first heart sound was replaced by a loud blowing systolic murmur with no opening snap, and he was fibrillating. At post mortem he was found to have multiple cerebral emboli.

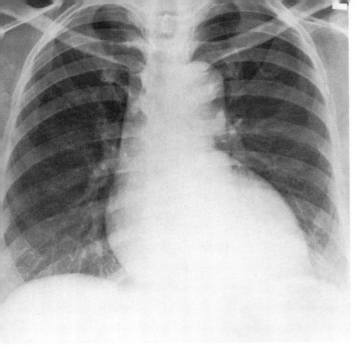

Figure 134   MRS. BABCOCK AGE 43

FOUR PATIENTS ADMITTED TO MEDICINE FROM THE CLINIC

Are the following **Roentgen Findings** present on any of these films?

One-liter pleural effusion.

Prominent aortic knob.

Widened aorta, both ascending and descending.

Calcification which could be pericardial.

Engorged hilar vessels and increased vascular markings.

Pronounced cardiac enlargement.

Rotation off the sagittal plane.

Valid mediastinal shift.

Dilated superior vena cava.

Convex left cardiac border.

Missing rib.

The **Historical Items** below *might* be appropriate to which?

Sudden chest pain and dyspnea, three hours.

Pulsatile headaches three months.

Heart murmur since childhood.

Back pain and hematuria.

Abdominal swelling without ankle edema.

Rheumatic fever at age 10.

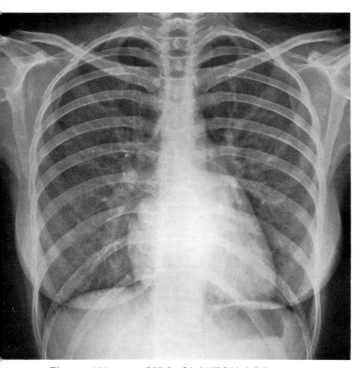

Figure 135   MRS. CLAYTON AGE 24

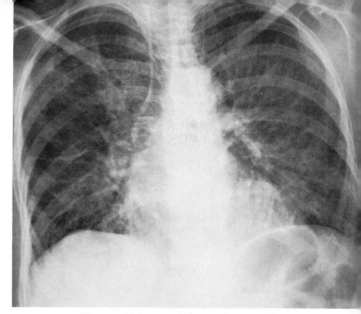

Figure 136　　　MR. ARCHER AGE 51

The following **Physical Signs** could fit which?

BP 230/110 both arms and even higher in both legs.

Markedly increased venous pressure of 35.

Presystolic murmur.

Quiet heart with decreased amplitude of pulsations at fluoroscopy.

Fibrillation.

Hepatomegaly.

Ankle edema.

Dyspnea on exertion.

Dyspnea at rest.

EKG shows low voltage QRS complexes.

EKG normal.

EKG shows notched P waves.

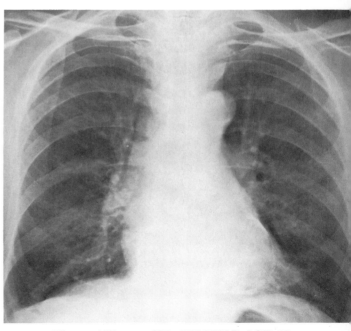

Figure 137　　　MR. BELKNAP AGE 46

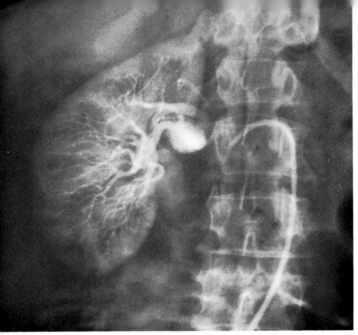

Figure 138   MRS. BABCOCK

ANSWERS

Renal Hypertension

Mrs. Babcock had hypertension of 230/110 and very severe headaches which had developed within a period of three months. She also complained of right back pain and had some microscopic hematuria. Her intravenous urogram was not definitely abnormal, but the selective renal angiogram (Fig. 138) showed an aneurysm of the right renal artery which was revised surgically with remission of the hypertension. Her chest film shows cardiac enlargement with a prominent left ventricle and a generally widened aorta. She was not in failure.

Rheumatic Heart Disease

Mrs. Clayton had had rheumatic fever in childhood and had always known she had a murmur. She, too, had back pain and hematuria and was thought to have cast a renal embolus. She was fibrillating and had classic murmurs for MS and MI. Her film shows, besides the convex left heart border, an elevated left main bronchus and the dense shadow of the left atrium seen through the heart and projecting to the right.

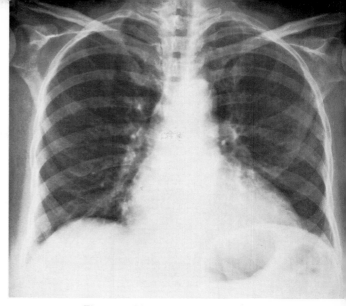

Figure 139   MR. ARCHER

Myocardial Infarction in Acute Congestive Failure

Mr. Archer has engorged hilar and pulmonary vessels. He presented about four hours after onset of acute chest pain and was dyspneic at rest. The EKG was normal at the time this film was made, but by the time the failure had responded to therapy and Figure 139 was made the EKG indicated a recent myocardial infarction. His liver was never down and he had no ascites. His film is rotated off the sagittal plane and the aorta is slightly unrolled; hence, the suggestion of mediastinal shift must be discounted.

Constrictive Pericarditis

Mr. Belknap has calcification about the heart in two projections, implying that it must be diffusely distributed in a shell encasing the ventricles. (Figure 140 is his lateral; there are traces of barium in the esophagus not to be mistaken for part of the calcification.) He presented with ascites without ankle edema, hepatomegaly, dyspnea on exertion only, and distended neck veins. His superior vena cava appears distended on the chest film and his systemic venous pressure was elevated. A diagnosis of constrictive pericarditis was confirmed at surgery. (Although calcification of the pericardium does not necessarily imply constriction, the syndrome of constriction *is* very common in patients with large amounts of calcium.)

Nobody has a missing rib or pleural effusion. Episodes with effusion would be anticipated, however, in any of these patients.

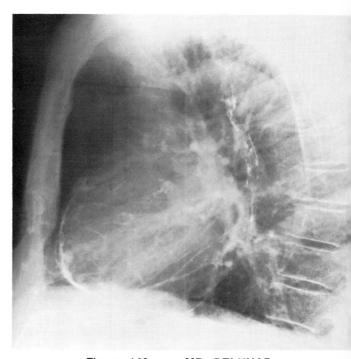

Figure 140   MR. BELKNAP

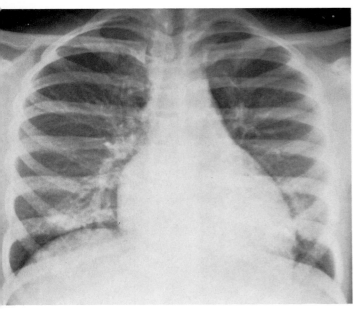

Figure 141   MR. DUANE

Figure 142   MR. DUANE

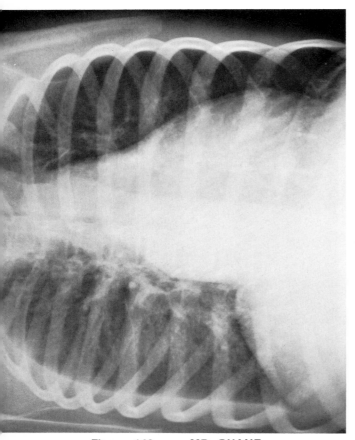

Figure 143   MR. DUANE

RECONCILING CONFLICTING ROENTGEN EVIDENCE

In this exercise you have two patients whose various films have to be reconciled with each other *because roentgen evidence is conflicting.* Which pieces of evidence are most convincing and how can you explain others that do not seem to agree with them?

Figure 143 must be interpreted at variance with Figures 141 and 142 — why?

Figure 145 belies the pathology at first suggested by Figure 144 — why?

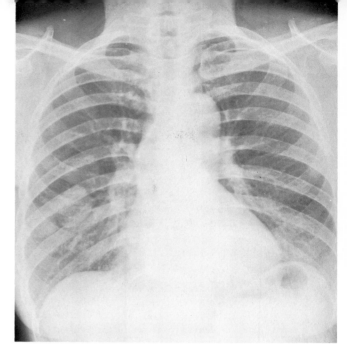

Figure 144   MRS. ABERNATHY

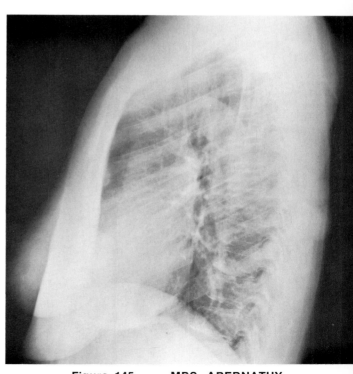

Figure 145   MRS. ABERNATHY

ANSWERS

Mr. Duane's diaphragms are at the eighth rib on his PA film and you may have been tempted to discount his cardiac enlargement for that reason. Perhaps you noted that in the lateral film the top of the stomach bubble is quite distant from the dome of the left diaphragm; something must be occupying that space! There is no fluid whatever in the two sharp posterior angles on the lateral nor in the costo-phrenic sinuses in the PA view. However, the decubitus film *definitely* shows fluid separating lung from chest wall, indicating without any possible question the presence of pleural fluid. After a check to make certain all three films were made on the same patient (they were) you must conclude that the right diaphragmatic shadows in the PA and lateral films are actually fluid imprisoned underneath the lung and above the diaphragm. The patient was going into failure and had had several other attacks of cardiac insufficiency.

Mrs. Abernathy shows several sharply margined nodules in the right lung field below the level of the hilum. Examination of the lung area on the lateral film fails to reveal anything to correspond with their size and shape. After checking the unit numbers to make sure this is indeed her lateral chest film, you restudy the film more closely and note the knobby appearance of the soft tissues of the back. Examination of the patient herself reveals three superficial neurofibromas below the right scapula

In studying radiographs you must realize that *all* the roentgen findings have to be reconciled to your satisfaction. Apparent inconsistencies may sometimes be explained as technical, may sometimes result in the un-scrambling of mislabeled films, and at other times may lead to a closer study of the films at hand and a diagnostic possibility not previously entertained.

SPECIAL EXERCISE
(NO FILMS)

What would be your conclusion if each of the following patients had had a single, perfectly normal PA chest film made at deep inspiration yesterday?

1. A man of 50 with an EKG showing evidence of a recent posterior myocardial incident of some importance.

2. A woman of 25 with bright red hemoptysis twice in the past week, and a dry cough.

3. A man who has coughed for years without fever or loss of weight and raises a half cup of sputum every morning.

4. A man with periodic chest pain which radiates down his left arm.

5. A child who has coughed and wheezed since yesterday when he choked on some popcorn.

6. A man of 60 who coughs, has lost 15 pounds in weight, and says he has had pneumonia twice in the past three months.

ANSWERS

A knowledge of the limitations of the roentgen method of investigation of disease is as important as an acquaintance with its helpful positive findings.

1. A posterior myocardial infarction may not give rise to any change in the efficiency of the heart function, and the chest film could remain normal throughout the episode.

2. Bright red hemoptysis and cough may indicate early active tuberculosis which is still invisible on the PA chest film. It may also go with a bronchial adenoma in a young woman, or, of course, any other cause of bleeding in the upper respiratory tract.

3. The history suggests bronchiectasis which is usually hard to visualize on plain films of the chest without the special procedure, bronchography.

4. Coronary insufficiency and anginal pain may be associated with a normal cardiac configuration on the chest film, though it is more commonly would show some cardiomegaly.

5. Nonopaque foreign bodies may act as ball valves, obstructing the egress but not the ingress of air through one main bronchus. There is frequently a stage at which the mediastinum is in the midline at full inspiration though it deviates far to the uninvolved side with each expiration. Hence, a single film made at inspiration may be entirely normal.

6. Bronchogenic carcinoma may cause repeated episodes of atelectasis, sometimes mistaken for pneumonia.

FOUR PATIENTS WITH MEDIASTINAL MASSES

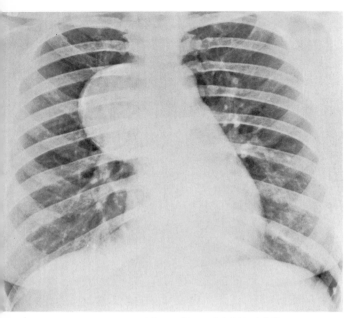

Figure 146   MRS. DAVIDSON AGE 32

Mrs. Davidson consults you because of a cough without fever for three weeks, headaches brought on by smelling bacon cooking, an aching pain in her left knee at night, and attacks of nausea and vomiting whenever her husband calls her from his mother's apartment where he goes once a week for dinner. On being asked whether her cough yields any sputum, she insists that from time to time she has coughed up red hair. She is very good looking with red hair, blue eyes, and very white skin.

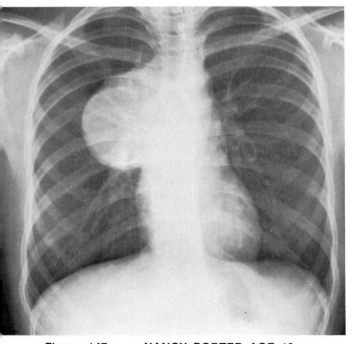

Figure 147   NANCY PORTER AGE 10

Nancy Porter is brought in by her parents who are worried because she wakes up at night crying and complaining of back pain. This usually happens after an active day and has been going on for about two years, but a careful check up had been entirely negative a year ago at the Army Base where Sgt. Porter was stationed.

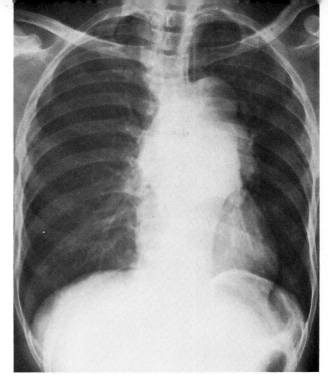

Mr. Rankin, too, consults you because of back pain, more or less constant, throbbing in character and localized to the midthoracic spine.

Figure 148   **MR. RANKIN AGE 50**

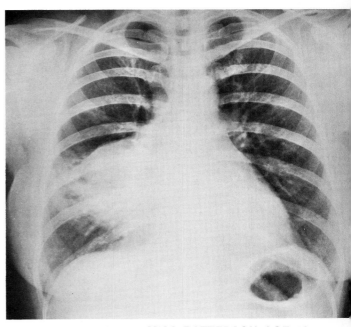

Miss Patterson has no complaints but has asked for a general physical exam prior to taking on several years of graduate study during which she will have to work days and go to school nights.

Figure 149   **MISS PATTERSON AGE 29**

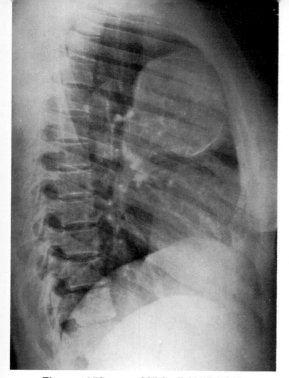

Figure 150   MRS. DAVIDSON

ANSWERS

Mrs. Davidson's left lateral film is Figure 150. She has a mediastinal mass which must be anterior because it clearly ablates the border of heart and aorta. This proved to be a dermoid cyst, and it contained red hair, all of which goes to show that you should listen to the patient; he is telling you what is wrong with him and there *may* be one significant bit of information in the middle of an improbable tale.

Nancy Porter has a mediastinal mass, but the border of the ascending aorta may be seen through the mass. The hilar vessels can be seen superimposed on it, which always tells you the mass is not in the hilum but in front of or behind it. There is another finding of great importance: the medial portion of the posterior sixth rib is missing, suggesting bone erosion which should also, of course, place the tumor far posterior in the chest. Note that the lateral (Fig. 151) confirms this, and that an AP bucky detail (Fig. 154) shows erosion of ribs and vertebral bodies. Posterior mediastinal masses are most commonly neural in origin, and in young girls very frequently ganglioneuromas, the final operative diagnosis in Nancy.

Mr. Rankin has a posterior mediastinal mass, too, which seems to produce not only a bulge in the descending aorta (follow its lateral margin upward from the diaphragm) and widening of the aortic knob, but also a dense white shadow seen through the heart. In the lateral (Fig. 153) this again seems to be a part of the aorta and clearly erodes the anterior margins of two thoracic vertebrae. Figure 152, his angiogram, proves that the mass is vascular and an aortic aneurysm.

Miss Patterson has a dermoid cyst, again in the anterior mediastinum. It was removed surgically and contained fatty material.

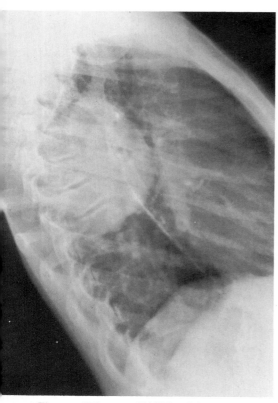

Figure 151   NANCY PORTER

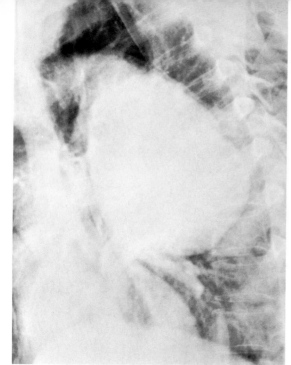

Figure 152   MR. RANKIN

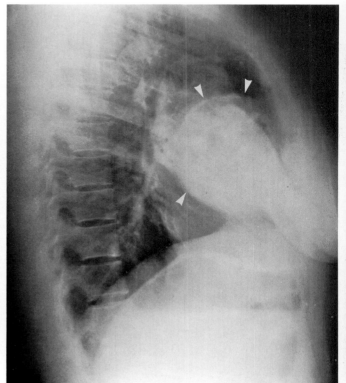

Figure 153   MR. RANKIN

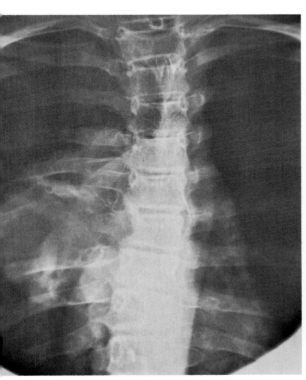

Figure 154   NANCY PORTER

Figure 155   MISS PATTERSON

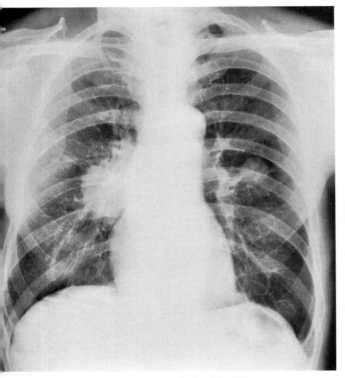

Figure 156　　MR. ASTOR

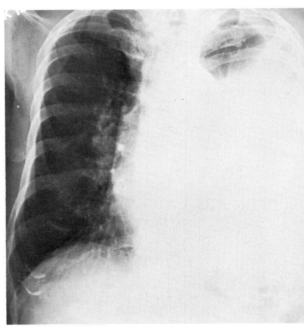

Figure 157　　MR. NASH

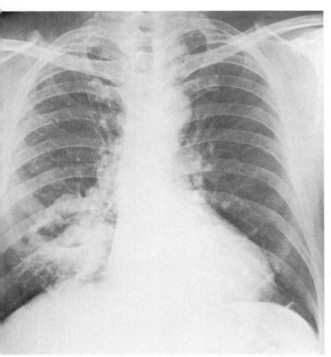

Figure 158　　MR. IRELAND

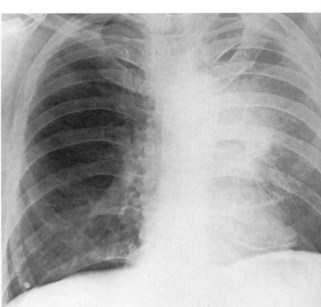

Figure 159　　MR. CASPER

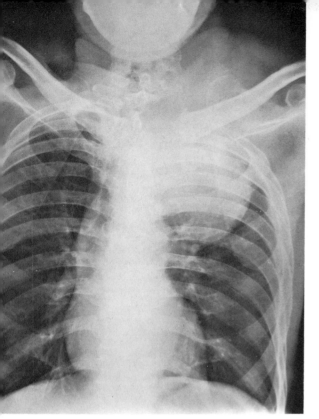

Figure 160   MR. ROGERS

SIX MEN WITH CHEST SYMPTOMS

Follow directions precisely

First (1) study the films carefully and note all **roentgen findings** you can be certain of before reading any farther.

Then (2) try to decide what symptoms each man reported to his doctor.

Then (3) tally the particular nine roentgen findings listed below with the initial of the appropriate patient's last name (zero if none fits).

And finally (4) decide what disease entity *could* have been the final pathological diagnosis in all six men.

SPECIFIC ROENTGEN FINDINGS

_____ EROSION RIGHT POSTERIOR SEVENTH RIB

_____ MEDIASTINAL SHIFT TO THE LEFT

_____ EROSION OF RIBS AND VERTEBRAE

_____ THICK-WALLED ABSCESS SUGGESTING BROKEN-DOWN TUMOR

_____ BILATERAL SUPERIOR MEDIASTINAL WIDENING

_____ EVIDENCE OF COLLAPSE OF AN ENTIRE LUNG

_____ HYDROTHORAX WITHOUT PNEUMOTHORAX

_____ EVIDENCE FOR LEFT UPPER LOBE COLLAPSE

_____ DISSEMINATED PULMONARY MASSES

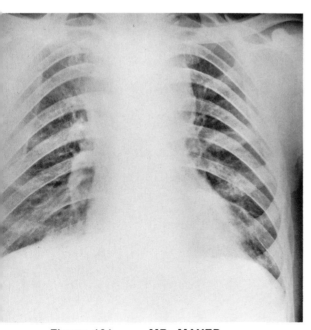

Figure 161   MR. MAYER

ANSWERS

You should have a nice sense of satisfaction on completing the foregoing exercise. Hopefully it has proved to you how much radiology you have learned. The tallying of a few of the specific roentgen findings present on these six chest films will have provided you with the word **Acrimonca,** a vertical (*scrambled*) acrostic of **Carcinoma,** the final diagnosis in all six patients.

Lung cancer has so wide a spectrum of roentgen findings and so varied a pattern of presenting complaints that it affords teachers of radiology a superb opportunity for review, not only of radiology but also of the pathophysiology of the disease.

All six patients had cough of some duration and weight loss. Only *Mr. Ireland's* cough was productive of much sputum, although both *Mr. Rogers* and *Mr. Casper* had had hemoptysis several times.

Mr. Astor and *Mr. Rogers* presented with back pain. *Mr. Astor's* pain was below the right scapula, sometimes radiating around to the front, and he was at first believed to have herpes zoster.

Mr. Rogers' pain was classic for lung cancer when it occurs close to the apex of the upper lobe (often called a Pancoast or superior sulcus tumor) and involves the brachial plexus. His pain was in the left shoulder and arm and he himself was concerned he might have angina. His film shows erosion of the posterior segments of the first three ribs and also of the left transverse processes and laminae of the first three thoracic vertebrae. (See Figure 162, a bucky detail of the thoracic inlet.)

Mr. Nash and *Mr. Casper* presented with dyspnea, and *Mr. Mayer* said he "could not get his breath." He had stridor audible across the room and the distended neck veins seen with

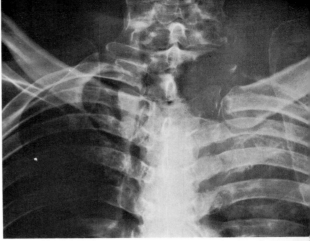

Figure 162   **BUCKY DETAIL — MR. ROGERS**

superior mediastinal syndrome. On examination he had a Horner's syndrome. His trachea and sympathetic chain were encircled by a mass of metastatic nodes and his primary is not visible but was in the right upper lobe bronchus. (Faced with this kind of mediastinal widening or symptoms suggestive of a Pancoast tumor, supplementary studies such as a bucky film, esophagram, laminagrams, and angiographic procedures are indicated.)

Mr. Nash had pleural seeding from the left lower lobe tumor you cannot see in the presence of so much pleural fluid. There were malignant cells in fluid taken during a diagnostic thoracentesis.

Mr. Casper had a carcinoma obstructing his left upper lobe bronchus and collapse of the lobe distal to the tumor as the imprisoned air was resorbed. There is little rotation, certainly not enough to explain the shift of both trachea and heart to the left. None of the left heart border is seen, which implies airless left upper lobe lying against it. The well visualized left diaphragm, on the other hand, tells you that the left lower lobe is inflated. (None of the six patients has roentgen evidence of collapse of a whole lung, of course.)

Mr. Astor has, in addition to his missing rib, a mass on the right and a smaller round mass in the left lung. His rib involvement is a lytic metastasis to bone rather than the erosion by contiguous extension of tumor you see in *Mr. Rogers*. The mass on the right was a primary bronchogenic carcinoma in the superior segment of the right lower lobe. (Note visible hilar vessels superimposed on it.) The mass in the left lung was a metastasis.

Of these six patients, only *Mr. Ireland* survived. His right lung and abscessed tumor were resected, and he was alive five years later without evidence of recurrence.

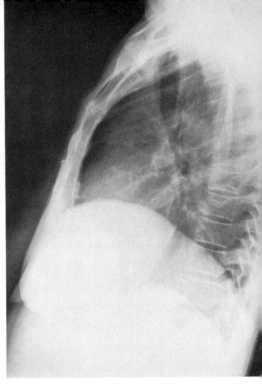

Figure 163

FINAL EXERCISE ON THE ANALYSIS OF THE LATERAL CHEST FILM

No names, no ages, no presenting symptoms, no clinical story, not even the related PA views! Just the laterals to compare and analyze. There are ten of them on this page spread and the next. Jot down your findings on a piece of paper before you look at the answers, since to commit yourself to paper is enormously more instructive than a cursory verbal commitment.

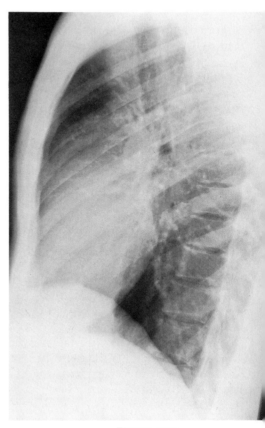

Figure 164

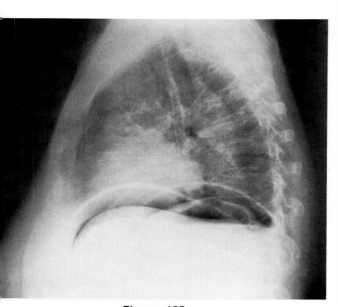

Figure 165

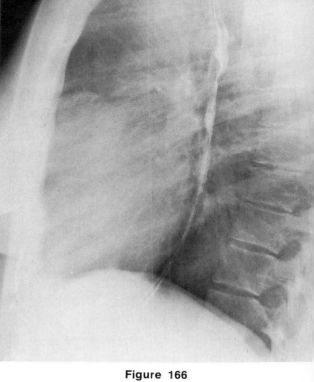

Figure 166

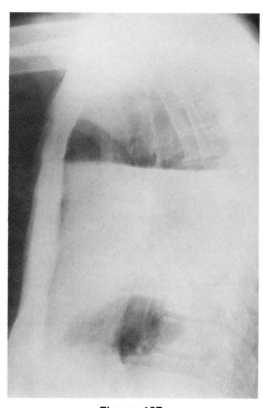

Figure 167

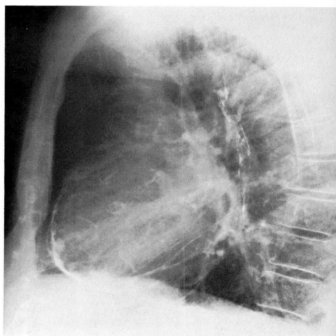

Figure 168

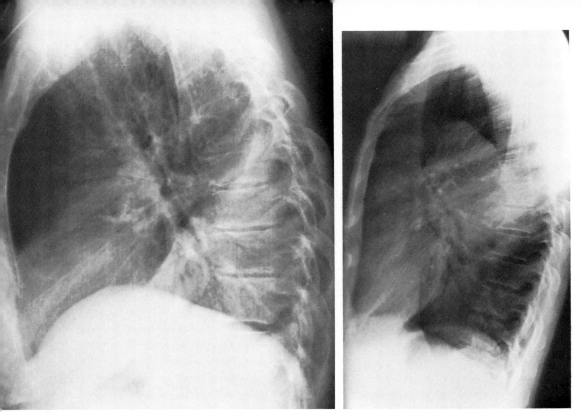

Figure 169

Figure 170

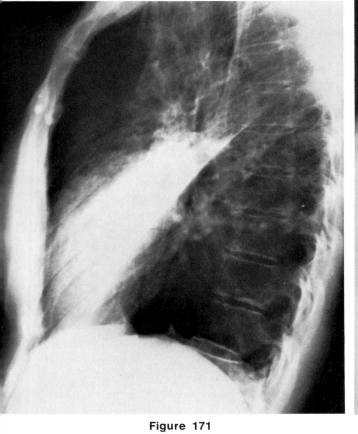

Figure 171

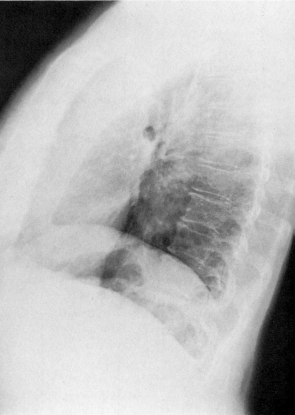

Figure 172

ANSWERS

Fig. 163: High right diaphragm, big liver with metastases from colon carcinoma (repeat of Fig. 19).

Fig. 164: Normal left lateral (repeat of Fig. 18).

Fig. 165: Free peritoneal air under both diaphragms (repeat of Fig. 30).

Fig. 166: Thymoma in the anterior mediastinum (repeat of Fig. 29).

Fig. 167: Left hydropneumothorax (repeat of Fig. 50).

Fig. 168: Pericardial calcification (repeat of Fig. 140).

Fig. 169: Left lower lobe pneumonia (repeat of Fig. 109).

Fig. 170: Aortic aneurysm (repeat of Fig. 153).

Fig. 171: Left upper lobe pneumonia (repeat of Fig. 153).

Fig. 172: Left upper lobe collapse (repeat of Fig. 112).

(NOTE: *Both students and teachers should realize that because the eye tends to recognize any given film when it is studied a second time, the student has been at an advantage in this exercise. However, with a large number of films the advantage is principally one of increased confidence, on the whole a good thing. Now try some laterals cold!)*

INDEX

DIAGNOSIS RELATED TO FIGURE NUMBERS